# Psychological Medicine

John Bancroft

The premenstrual syndrome – a reappraisal of the concept and the evidence

MONOGRAPH SUPPLEMENT 24

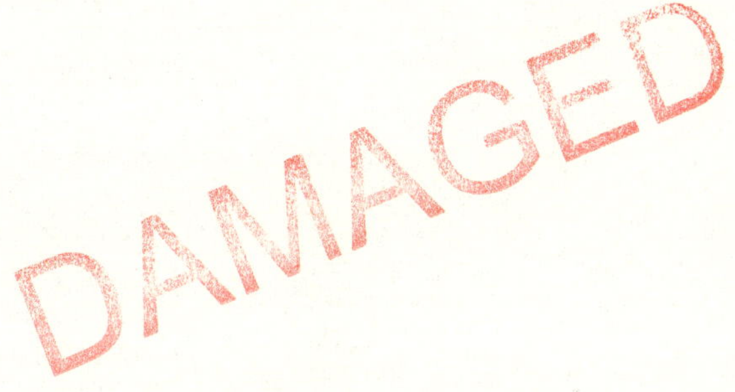


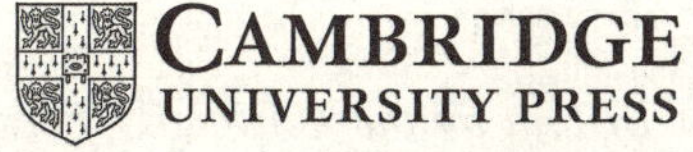
CAMBRIDGE
UNIVERSITY PRESS

PUBLISHED BY
THE PRESS SYNDICATE OF THE UNIVERSITY OF CAMBRIDGE

The Pitt Building, Trumpington Street, Cambridge CB2 1RP
40 West 20th Street, New York, N.Y. 10011–4211, U.S.A.
10 Stamford Road, Oakleigh, Melbourne 3166, Australia



*Printed in Great Britain by the University Press, Cambridge*

**CONTENTS**

List of Figures

I am indebted to Dr Cynthia Graham for her careful reading of the manuscript and for access to her extensive knowledge of the literature, without which my task would have been much harder. I am also grateful to Dr Rodney Kelly and Dr Peter Illingworth for their helpful comments.

SYNOPSIS   The Premenstrual Syndrome (PMS) remains a controversial issue. As a clinical concept it is surrounded by confusion. Attempts to establish a consensus definition have resulted in the majority of women seeking help for such problems excluded from the diagnosis. Furthermore, there is no consensus about how such problems should be treated, with a variety of methods being advocated usually on very uncertain scientific grounds. The issue also has its political implications; there are those who see PMS as a way of reducing the status of women, by linking the normal ovarian cycle to a phenomenon which, on the face of it, impairs women's ability to cope. Yet there are a substantial number of women who experience significant negative changes which vary with the menstrual cycle, and produce long-term effects on their well being and family relationship which can be serious. There is also a real possibility that recurrent perimenstrual mood changes of this kind may increase the likelihood of chronic depressive illness in susceptible individuals. In most respects the features of depression which occurs perimenstrually are essentially similar to those of major depressive disorder, except for the short duration and recurrent pattern.

PMS, therefore, remains an issue not only of clinical importance, but of considerable potential relevance to our understanding of major depressive disorder, which is substantially more common in women of reproductive age than in their male counterparts.

In this review the concept of PMS, and some prominent operational definitions of it, are critically evaluated; it is now questionable whether the concept, as currently applied, still carries any heuristic or clinical value. Some current theoretical and aetiological issues are considered: e.g. the role of the corpus luteum, the effects of hormonal regimes which block ovulation, such as oral contraceptives, and the possibility that cyclical mood change represents an entrained rhythm in the brain.

The conclusions reached at this stage in the review lead to a 'paradigm shift' with the proposal of a three-factor model to account for the complexities of menstrual cycle-related problems. These three factors are (a) the 'timing factor', imposed by the ovarian hormonal cycle, and possibly accounting for cyclical changes in CNS neurotransmitter activity; (b) a 'menstruation factor', including the processes involved in the build up as well as shedding of the endometrium and the ways in which these processes might adversely affect the women's well being both premenstrually as well as during menstruation; and (c) the 'vulnerability factor', covering a variety of characteristics, constitutional as well as situational, psychosocial as well as biological, which are not in themselves functions of the menstrual cycle but which serve to determine how vulnerable a woman will be to the first two factors.

The relevant evidence in the literature is then reappraised according to this reformulation. Although important questions remain unanswered, many crucial issues start to look less confusing and a more obvious research agenda suggests itself. The political issue is also 'defused'; the variability of well being which commonly accompanies the ovarian cycle is unlikely, on its own, to lead to significant problems unless it interacts with other factors, most of which are as likely to lead to difficulty in men as in women.

Address for correspondence: Dr John Bancroft, MRC Reproductive Biology Unit, Royal Edinburgh Hospital, Morningside Park, Edinburgh EH10 5HF.

# I. INTRODUCTION

The premenstrual syndrome remains a controversial issue. Clinically, there is prevailing confusion about how it should be treated and as a consequence, considerable scope for exploitation of those seeking treatment. Politically, there are many in the women's movement who see this as one of the more striking examples of medicalization of women's health, as well as fuel for those who prefer to see women as more vulnerable and hence less reliable than men.

Yet behind this controversy is a clinical problem of some magnitude. For whatever reason, there are many women who suffer considerable distress which they see as related to their menstrual cycles. The concept of premenstrual syndrome (PMS) has offered many of them a hope of relief which all too often leads to disappointment. The problem also has wider implications because of a possible link with depressive illness in women. The need to improve our understanding of this problem is therefore substantial.

Clinical researchers working in the field have increasingly come to recognize that the concept, as it has prevailed, is flawed and that some form of reformulation is required. Some with both a biological (e.g. Rubinow & Schmidt, 1992) and a feminist (e.g. Ussher, 1992) approach to the problem have offered alternative strategies for tackling the complexity of the problem. This review also aims to scrutinize critically the concept of PMS and to offer a re-formulation in an attempt to provide a constructive way forward.


# II. DEFINITION

It has frequently been stated that the primary reason for the inconclusive, often conflicting research findings in this area has been the lack of an agreed definition of PMS (e.g. Magos & Studd, 1984; Rubinow *et al.* 1985; Reid, 1986). According to Dalton (1984) 'the failure to adhere to the strict definition of premenstrual syndrome has resulted in confusion and consequently has produced conflicting results' (p. 4). An alternative view is that the confusion has resulted principally from the need to create a single diagnostic category to cover a very wide range of phenomena, having in common only their temporal relationship to the menstrual cycle. Attempts at definition have sought to impose arbitrary criteria which may have served to obscure key characteristics and delay our proper understanding of the varied phenomena in question. From this viewpoint, the problem has not been a lack of an agreed definition but a failure to identify satisfactorily what it is that requires to be defined. In the fullness of time the history of PMS may well serve as an example of how the need for a discrete medical diagnosis can obscure clinical reality.

Because we see this conceptual issue as fundamental to the whole subject, we will consider some of the attempts to arrive at a definition in detail.

Dalton has been one of the leading exponents of the concept of 'premenstrual syndrome'. Her definition is brief – 'Premenstrual syndrome is the recurrence of symptoms in the premenstruum with absence of symptoms in the post-menstruum' (Dalton, 1984, p. 3) – and is solely dependent on the timing of symptoms and not on their character. 'Definitively, the premenstruum covers the four days immediately before menstruation; these are the days of greatest severity of symptoms in premenstrual syndrome...' For diagnosis of the condition she asserts that 'symptoms must be relieved by the onset of full menstrual flow' (p. 10). However, elsewhere she concedes that 'symptoms that have started during the premenstruum may continue during the first few days of menstruation' (p. 4), and further 'when it was realised that the recurring symptoms were at their peak during the last 4 days of the premenstruum and the first 4 days of menstruation it became necessary to find a word to cover these vital 8 days – paramenstruum'.

However, she does not refer to the 'para-menstrual syndrome'.

Let us look more closely at her definition.

1. It is based solely on timing, but the concept of time shifts from statement to statement. Applying her definition logically, any woman whose symptoms reached their peak 5 days prior to the onset of menstrual bleeding or during menstruation would not be included, even though they might show a recurring cyclical pattern. It requires a particular type of temporal pattern, although she acknowledges that various temporal patterns occur. She does not explain why only those conforming to her temporal pattern justify membership of this category while other cyclical patterns are excluded.

2. It is not concerned with the type, number or severity of symptoms. This reflects the recognition that a wide range of experiences are reported by women to vary through the menstrual cycle. Any of these, including acne, eczema, breast tenderness, irritable bowel, backache, urinary frequency, nausea, hot flushes, could constitute her syndrome so defined.

3. It is dependent on the 'absence of symptoms for at least 7 days'. What in operational terms does this mean? There are certain types of symptom, e.g. headaches, which are either present or absent, and to which such a definition might be applied. But a symptom such as irritability is part of normal experience, ranging in degree according to circumstances as well as temperament. Is a women to be 'free from irritability' for at least 7 days before she can be put into this category? It is noteworthy that Dalton uses a binary system for recording symptoms; they are either present or absent. The scope for distortion or bias with such a system is considerable. Most others in the field attempt some form of grading of severity.

Although Dalton's requirement of a symptom-free phase is highly questionable, some form of timing requirements, along her lines, are commonplace in the many definitions that have been offered. As Vergare (1987) pointed out 'The cessation of symptoms with or shortly after the onset of menses is used to differentiate premenstrual syndrome from the broader spectrum of menstrual related disorders' (p. 215). Interestingly, this 'broader spectrum' has received scant attention, as we shall see later.

Moving on to other definitions, Reid (1985) offered the following: 'The cyclical recurrence, in the luteal phase of the menstrual cycle, of any combination of distressing physical, psychological and/or behavioural changes of sufficient severity to result in deterioration of interpersonal relationships and/or interference with normal activities' (p. 5). Here we have a timing criterion which is possibly more problematical, in operational terms, than Dalton's; a recurrence during the luteal phase (i.e. approximately half of the cycle), but no indication whether this should be confined to the luteal phase, or should start or finish within it. This definition introduces another dimension – severity. What is the purpose of severity criteria? Clearly, they are useful in order to assess the prevalence of a problem of clinical significance, and necessary for the selection of subjects for treatment studies. But they may also serve as an impediment for research into the origins and determinants of cycle-related phenomena. Any criterion of severity is bound to be arbitrary; it will not in any sense discriminate between different aetiologies. Rubinow (1987) pointed out that by using severity criteria, avoidance or at least reduction of the misleading effects of attribution would result, as these are likely to be less influential in severe cases. That may be so, but there are counterbalancing disadvantages. By requiring severe distress or disruption, other variables are introduced which will be unrelated in any direct sense to the phenomenon under investigation but rather reflect non-specific personality characteristics related to 'tolerance of discomfort', or patterns of help-seeking behaviour. As we shall see later, such factors are likely to be highly relevant to the clinical situation but of uncertain relevance to the basic aetiology.

Haskett *et al.* (1980) offered a more complex but also more sophisticated definition, or 'set of diagnostic criteria'. They examined a number of women presenting with 'perimenstrual complaints' and first assessed which types of complaints were most common. This led them to list a number of types of symptom without which the diagnosis of what they called 'Primary Recurrent Premenstrual Tension Disorder' should not be made:

(*a*) at least five of eight sets of mood and behavioural symptoms;

(*b*) overall disturbance is so severe that at least

one of the following is present: (i) serious impairment socially, with family, at home, at school or work; or, (ii) sought, or was referred for help, or took medication;

(*c*) premenstrual dysphoric symptoms for at least six of the nine preceding menstrual cycles;

(*d*) symptoms *only during the premenstrual period with relief soon after onset of menses.*

This definition introduces criteria involving the type of symptoms, with particular emphasis on emotional or affective changes. The term used involves 'tension'; a woman with severe and recurrent breast tenderness or bloating would not qualify for this diagnosis. Other investigators have criticized this definition on the grounds that it fails to account for the diversity of symptoms and describes only a narrow-based, single syndrome (Halbreich & Endicott, 1985*a*). Another criticism relates to their requirement that symptoms be present for at least *six* of the last nine cycles; the considerable inter-cycle variability in symptom severity that has been demonstrated (Hart *et al.* 1987) makes this criterion overly stringent.

In a controversial appendix to the proposed revision of the Diagnostic and Statistical Manual of Mental Disorders or DSM-III-R (DSM-III-R, 1987), the term Late Luteal Phase Dysphoric Disorder was introduced, to provide a systematic set of diagnostic criteria for a premenstrual mood disorder. This diagnosis requires that at least five of 10 symptoms (*at least one affective in nature*) be present for 'most of the time during each symptomatic late luteal phase'. Additional requirements are that symptoms: (*a*) be present 'in most menstrual cycles during the past year'; (*b*) remit 'within a few days after onset of the follicular phase'; (*c*) seriously interfere with work or with usual social activities or relationships with others'; and, (*d*) are not merely 'an exacerbation of the symptoms of another disorder, such as Major Depression, Panic Disorder, Dysthymia or a Personality Disorder'. Lastly, a definite diagnosis can only be made if the symptoms are confirmed by prospective daily self-ratings of symptoms during at least two symptomatic cycles.

The term Late Luteal Phase Dysphoric Disorder (LLPDD) emphasizes the assumed link with the corpus luteum of the ovarian cycle, reflecting the widely held belief that this 'phenomenon' only occurs during ovulatory cycles. (We will return to this belief later.) This definition does not specify any degree of change or severity criteria. In a recent study which utilized five different change criteria and compared women meeting criteria for LLPDD with a control group of women without premenstrual complaints, none of these change criteria differentiated the two groups, making the diagnosis of LLPDD problematical (Gallant *et al.* 1992).

Although definitions of PMS have increased in complexity, they have not improved in operational quality. For the most part, while they can be used simply for clinical purposes, they are of little value for research purposes because of the vague nature of so many of the 'essential' requirements. For example, in the LLPDD definition, symptoms must have been present 'most of the time' during the late luteal phase and have remited 'within a few days after onset of the follicular phase'.

In an effort to establish operational criteria to define a cycle-related mood disorder, an NIMH-sponsored workshop (National Institute of Mental Health, 1983) suggested a 30% change in mood during the week before menstruation as compared with the week following cessation of menses in two of three cycles. These guidelines have been adopted in a number of studies, although recently their utility has been questioned. Gallant *et al.* (1992) have suggested that the 30% criterion of change may be non-discriminative in that they apply to women who do not report significant premenstrual changes. On the other hand, these criteria would also exclude cases in which the 30% increase was evident but only when the last 4 premenstrual and first 3 menstrual days were averaged.

When we turn to those research studies which set out to establish what type of cyclical patterns occur and with what frequency, we find some interesting variations on the theme which has already emerged. Thus, Magos *et al.* (1986*a*) started off with a commendably open definition of 'premenstrual syndrome' – 'Distressing physical, psychological and behavioural symptoms, not caused by organic disease, *which recur regularly during the same phase of each menstrual (or ovarian) cycle*, and which significantly regress or disappear during the remainder of the cycle' (p. 274, my italics). They went on to use Trend Analysis, a technique employing exponentially smoothed averages, to identify both the timing of peaks and troughs and whether they digressed significantly from the mean. This offered an appropriate method for establishing just what types of cyclical patterns occurred, and whether they were similar for different symptoms, and showed predictable timing across cycles. However, after this admirable start, these authors then found it necessary to impose some concept of PMS on their analysis, their definition changing to include 'significant ($P < 0.05$) positive symptom trends (i.e. peaks) at some time during the 14 days before menstruation and *at no other time during the cycle*, and significant negative symptom trends *at some time after the onset of menstruation and at no time after the presence of significant positive trends*' (my italics). They applied their method and this definition to 150 women who had described themselves as PMS sufferers (Magos *et al.* 1986*a*). They found that from 61 to 85% of women conformed to their definition of premenstrual syndrome, while 14 to 35% showed significant trends (i.e. 'cyclical' patterns) which did not conform. The varying percentages reflected the different symptoms that were examined. They called these two groups 'PMS + ve' and 'PMS − ve'. From 0 to 5% showed no significant trends. The 'PMS + ve' trends involved both physical and psychological symptoms, and the main difference from the 'PMS − ve' group, apart from the timing, was that in the latter group the principal symptoms showing the trends were varieties of negative affect, and there was less contrast between the peaks and troughs of these symptoms (i.e. less resolution). They therefore suggested that 'the primary difference between these two groups... may lie in the greater chronic morbidity manifested by those whose symptom profiles do not fulfil the diagnostic criteria for premenstrual syndrome rather than in the severity of the premenstrual symptoms' (p. 281). They concluded that 'the finding that the majority of women with premenstrual syndrome trends show premenstrual exacerbation for physical, psychological and behavioural parameters on a similar time scale, suggests that irrespective of symptoms, the primary aetiological mechanism for the syndrome is similar in all cases' (p. 281). Given their other findings, the illogicality of this statement is obvious. Perhaps a more appropriate conclusion might have been

'whereas, in the majority of cases, the peaks of physical and emotional symptoms occurred during the premenstrual phase of the cycle, there was a substantial proportion of women in whom the peaks of emotional symptoms were somewhat later and which showed less complete resolution. The explanation for this difference is not yet clear'.

In a further striking example of the imposition of an arbitrary definition, Hammarbäck *et al.* (1989) described their 'ideal' form of PMS in which symptoms develop only during the luteal phase of the cycle, and abate at the onset of the menstrual period disappearing by the third or fourth day of the cycle. They then used statistical techniques to establish the extent to which women's symptoms deviated from this ideal and how much of variation could be attributed to chance. In a series of 80 PMS clinic attenders, 30% qualified for 'pure PMS', 56% for 'premenstrual aggravation' and 14% as 'no significant cyclicity'. Once again, we are confined to a definition which arbitrarily specifies which phases of the menstrual cycle should show the peak and trough of the cyclical pattern. The precise nature of the large proportion who did not meet the strict criteria is not described.

In an enterprising study (Hurt *et al.* 1992), data were gathered together from 5 clinical centres in the US, resulting in daily ratings over two cycles for a total of 670 women. The emphasis of the study was to establish the incidence of Late Luteal Phase Dysphoric Disorder, as defined in DSM-III-R. They applied four different procedures to this data, the 'absolute severity' method, the 'per cent change' method (Eckerd *et al.* 1989), the 'effect size' method (Schnurr, 1989) and the 'trend analysis' method, as described above. The number of women meeting the criteria for LLPDD varied from 14%, using the 'absolute severity' method, to 45% with the 'trend analysis' method. The authors concluded that their results 'underscore the need for a uniform assessment method', but they did not comment on whether such a method should produce a high or a low proportion. Considering that all the subjects had been attending PMS clinics, it would be of interest to know how many of the women who did not meet these particular criteria showed cyclicity of other kinds.

Only a sample of the definitions of PMS

which have been proposed in recent years has been considered. My argument is that, by excluding a large number of women who show symptom patterns which do not fit an 'ideal' form of PMS, all of these definitions have served to limit the information we have on the different patterns of cycle-related changes women experience.

Arguments about the advantages and disadvantages of methods of classification of illness, or diagnosis, are by no means confined to those related to the menstrual cycle. Such controversy has been particularly strong in the general field of mental illness, and periodically the abandonment of diagnosis, or at least the focussing on symptoms rather than diagnostic categories, is advocated (e.g. Costello, 1992). But as Kendell (1975) has argued, diagnostic or classificatory systems do have important functions, several of which are germane to this discussion. Without some method of summarizing key features which some patients have in common it is difficult to plan the operational requirements for clinical care, or to carry out epidemiological studies which might throw light on important causative factors. The use of an appropriate diagnosis should clarify treatment. Indeed, for all the shortcomings of current psychiatric diagnosis, it can be argued that it enhances the efficacy with which modern methods of treatment are employed and evaluated. Unfortunately, no such benefit can properly be attributed to the diagnosis of 'premenstrual syndrome', however it is defined (claims to the contrary notwithstanding). The approach to treatment remains as confused as ever, compounded by the steady addition of alternative methods.

A further function of diagnostic classification is one which particularly concerns us in this review – the facilitation of research into aetiological mechanisms, which apart from its intrinsic interest might also lead to the improvement in treatment methods. The point that has been argued repeatedly about premenstrual syndrome, is that the underlying phenomenon does interact with other processes or illnesses to produce the confused picture which is often seen. Therefore, there are advantages in restricting research to examples of the 'pure culture' of premenstrual syndrome, even if such cases represent only a small proportion of those cases that come to clinician's attention. I do not disagree with this view. I would argue, however, that so far attempts to identify this 'pure form' have been confounded by the imposition of some preconceived concept, some 'social construct' of the key phenomenon. In other words, it is not simply that this particular diagnosis, however it has been operationally defined, has failed to help research into aetiology, it may actually have hindered it.

At this point, I would therefore advocate that, for both clinical and research purposes, no attempt should be made to define a condition called 'premenstrual syndrome'. Instead, we should identify cycle-related patterns of *specific symptoms* or changes (e.g. depression or food craving), with no preconceptions about their precise temporal relationship to menstruation or the ovarian cycle, but aiming to establish their tendency to recur across cycles, and with no assumptions about how these different cycle-related symptom patterns might relate to each other.

## III. AETIOLOGICAL MODELS

### A. The 'normal' ovarian cycle

The prevailing tendency has been to see PMS as a disorder of the ovarian cycle. Our understanding of the physiology of this fundamental cyclical phenomenon is far from complete, but the main features deserve a brief summary. The first day of menstrual bleeding is conventionally and arbitrarily regarded as the first day of a new cycle. This is the start of the follicular or proliferative phase; follicular because around this time a new follicle is selected to develop, producing increasing amounts of oestradiol; proliferative because the endometrium proliferates in response to the rising oestradiol. Selection of the dominant follicle is initiated by a brief intercycle rise in the concentration of the gonadotrophin, FSH, which thereafter drops in concentration during the follicular phase. The further development of the follicle is then maintained by FSH in association with LH, another gonadotrophin. LH stimulates the thecal cells of the ovarian stroma to secrete androgens, especially androstenedione; FSH stimulates the granulosa cells of the follicle to convert or aromatize the androgens into estradiol – $17\beta$. The circulating levels of this oestrogen rise gradually during this phase. FSH falls as

*J. Bancroft*

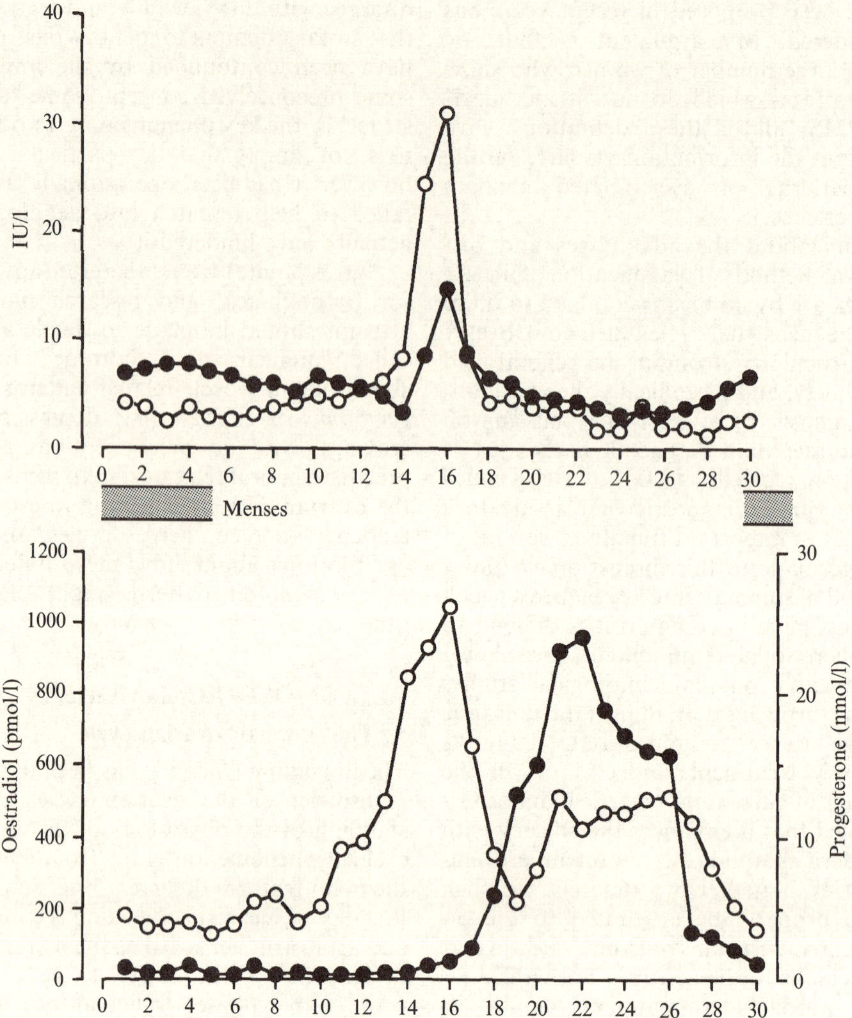

FIG. 1.   Mean daily levels of LH and FSH (top graph: ○, LH; ●, FSH) and progesterone and oestradiol (bottom graph: ○, oestradiol; ●, progesterone) through the cycle from four 'normal' women. The data are centred on the day of the LH peak. As the original cycle lengths varied, the timing of menstrual bleeding, as shown, is approximate. Note the different scales for progesterone and oestradiol. (Data derived, with permission, from Illingworth *et al.* 1990.)

a result of negative feedback; LH does not fall to the same extent and in fact, once the oestadiol reaches a certain level, shows a dramatic rise or surge which serves to induce ovulation – the release of the ovum from the ripened follicle. This LH surge is known as the 'positive feedback response' which is characteristic of the female's hypothalamo-pituary-gonadal axis and is central to the normal ovarian cycle. Following ovulation, the ruptured follicle becomes the corpus luteum and proceeds to secrete massive amounts of progesterone as well as further oestradiol (see Fig. 1). On a molar basis, the levels of progesterone attained are 100-fold higher than the oestradiol levels during the follicular phase. This second phase of the cycle is called the luteal phase, because of the activity of the corpus luteum, or the secretory phase, because of the added effects of the progesterone on endometrial development. The corpus luteum, however, has a limited life and in the absence of conception, it starts to regress (luteolysis) resulting in a fall of progesterone and oestradiol levels. This in turn is followed by the onset of endometrial shedding and menstrual bleeding, and the start of the next cycle.

Two events in this cycle, the switch from negative to positive feedback that proceeds the LH surge and ovulation, and luteal regression, are not well understood. The suprachiasmatic nucleus of the hypothalamus is involved in the regulation of the positive feedback response, as well as other biological rhythms. The main source of variation in the length of the ovarian cycle is the length of the follicular phase, which is largely determined by the timing of the 'intercycle' peak of FSH which initiates follicle selection and development. A variety of factors (e.g. stress, weight loss) can interfere with this process and either delay or prevent this FSH peak, in ways which are not understood. The length of the luteal phase is, by comparison, much more predictable: usually around 14 days, but varying from 11 to 17 days in otherwise normal cycles. Significant variations in luteal function (e.g. 'inadequate' or short luteal phases) may result from abnormalities in the pre-ovulatory LH surge.

Numerous attempts have been made to identify abnormalities of the ovarian cycle which distinguish PMS sufferers from non-sufferers. A recurring theme has been a search for differences in circulating levels of progesterone or the progesterone/oestradiol ratio during the luteal phase. No consistent findings have resulted. Other factors in the cycle have been examined in the same way. Such attempts have universally failed. I will not review this extensive and uninformative literature here. This has been done often enough before (Reid & Yen, 1981; Rausch & Janowsky, 1982; Bancroft & Bäckström, 1985; Rubinow & Schmidt, 1992). However, given the incompleteness of our understanding of the normal cycle and its control by the brain, and its inherent complexity, involving cascades of interacting homeostatic control mechanisms, such failure should not surprise us. The notion, that relevant abnormalities of such systems could be identified by occasional measurement of specific variables in the circulation of women with and without the so-called 'pre-menstrual syndrome', now seems exceptionally naive. At the very least we should have been looking for ways of testing or challenging the system.

More recently fresh attention has been drawn to the possible role of progesterone and its metabolites. MacDonald *et al.* (1991) stress not only the huge amounts of progesterone, compared to other steroids, that are secreted during the luteal phase, but also the bioactivity of some of its metabolites (e.g. the GABA activity of 5 alpha and beta reduced metabolites). They also postulate that the recurrence of ovulatory cycles in the modern premenopausal woman, who now experiences 'more than 450 episodes of massive progesterone secretion/withdrawal for physiologically futile purposes', may account for a variety of disorders 'that occur commonly but uniquely in women of reproductive age' (e.g. premenstrual syndrome and puerperal depression). It is questionable whether this shift in emphasis is likely to be helpful. It does take us away from the naive question of whether women with PMS have different circulating levels of progesterone to those without, and points out that there is variability among women in the total amount of progesterone secreted, and in the relative proportions of bioactive metabolites. It may therefore be of some interest to see whether such variations relate in any way to variations in premenstrual symptoms. But as yet we have negligible evidence deriving from this model. Rubinow & Schmidt (1992) compared the concentration of the GABA active metabolites, allopregnanolone and pregnanolone, in 15 women with PMS and 12 controls and found no differences. It remains to be seen whether this new line of enquiry will result in less naive research. But we will return to this issue later.

In the second part of this monograph we will confine our attention to a few key concepts that currently predominate in aetiological research. In particular we will consider: (*a*) the role of the corpus luteum, and (*b*) whether the cyclical variation in brain activity, which presumably underlies many of the symptoms, is a direct function of varying levels of ovarian hormones or rather an endogenous rhythm of brain activity which is temporally entrained by a 'biological clock' function of the ovarian cycle.

## B. The role of the corpus luteum

The recent American re-definition of the problem as Late Luteal Phase Dysphoric Disorder underlines the assumption that ovulation and the corpus luteum are prerequisites for 'PMS'. This assumption has been widespread. It has even been proposed that the presence of premenstrual symptoms is evidence that ovulation has occurred (Magyar *et al.* 1979). However, there have been few attempts to substantiate this assumption, and the issue remains uncertain though crucial.

Two early studies (Adamopoulos *et al.* 1972; Andersen *et al.* 1977) reported the occurrence of premenstrual symptoms during anovular cycles. In both the numbers involved were small and the criteria used to determine ovulation or the presence of premenstrual changes were not given. Bäckström *et al.* (1983) studied 55 women, 22 of whom complained of severe PMS. During monitoring, three women experienced 5 anovular cycles between them. During these cycles there was no evidence of cyclical mood change, although there was evidence of mild premenstrual breast tenderness. However, none of these women regarded herself as suffering from PMS.

Walker (1987) set out to recruit women who had an increased likelihood of experiencing anovular cycles i.e. women during the postpartum period or with irregular cycles associated with the perimenopause (when there is a substantially increased occurrence of anovular cycles; Metcalf, 1983). After a considerable recruitment effort, only three women with both ovular and anovular cycles were monitored. Apart from a tendency for premenstrual breast tenderness to be less noticeable in the anovular cycles, these pairs of cycles showed no more difference in symptom patterns than pairs of ovular cycles. However, once again the women involved were not experiencing clear patterns of premenstrual worsening in either cycle. Clearly this research approach, while of interest, is not an easy one to pursue.

The most substantial evidence comes from a study by Hammärback & Bäckström (1989). In a series of 124 women attending a PMS clinic, 8 women were found to have one ovulatory cycle, in which symptoms met the criteria of PMS (as previously discussed, see Hammarbäck *et al.* 1989), and one anovulatory cycle. Although two of these women showed cyclicity in one symptom during their anovular cycle ('depression' in one case, 'swelling' in the other), the anovular cycles were noticeably free from cyclical symptoms, compared with the ovular cycles. The authors concluded that the presence of a corpus luteum is involved in the development of cyclical symptoms. Though striking, these results raise further questions and cannot yet be regarded as conclusive. What caused the anovular cycles to occur? Is it possible that the reduction in premenstrual symptoms and the anovulation both resulted from the same factor, but one was not the consequence of the other? It is also noteworthy that, although a substantial proportion of the women in this study failed to meet the criteria of PMS in either one or both of the cycles monitored, there were no women with anovular cycles who failed to meet the criteria of PMS during an ovulatory cycle. Further evidence of this kind is required.

Apart from the absence of ovulation, other characteristics of the luteal phase are also germane to this discussion. What happens during cycles with either short or deficient luteal phases? Walker (1987) studied five women with one normal and one short luteal phase cycle, and four women with one normal and one inadequate luteal phase. Once again, in comparing these women with others showing two normal cycles, she found no suggestion that symptoms were of shorter duration or less intense in either type of abnormal cycle, although there was a tendency for breast tenderness to be less noticeable during the inadequate luteal phases. However, as for the women with anovular cycles in her study, these subjects were not experiencing 'PMS' in either normal or abnormal cycles. No other evidence of this kind has so far been reported.

We can pursue these questions further by looking at studies in which ovulation has been blocked either as an experimental procedure or as a consequence of a treatment method.

## C. The effects of oral contraceptives

The commonest method for blocking ovulation is the use of steroidal contraception. Most oral contraceptives (o.c.s) in current use contain a fixed dose of oestrogen and a progestagen, taken continuously for 21 days followed by a 7-day pill-free interval (the combined monophasic o.c.) The more recent, 'phasic' formulations contain a fixed dose of oestrogen combined with a graduated increase in progestagen, crudely mimicking the natural cycle.

In several early studies, it was reported that women using o.c.s were less likely to suffer from PMS, and beneficial effects of o.c.s on PMS were claimed (e.g. Grant & Pryse-Davies, 1968; Moos, 1968; Kutner & Brown, 1972). Moos (1969) concluded that there 'was little doubt that progestagen and estrogen combinations relieve a number of symptoms associated with pre-menstrual tension'. However, he added that in a proportion of women premenstrual symptoms were aggravated by o.c.s, leading him to suggest that women whose premenstrual symptoms were helped and those whose symptoms were aggravated by o.c.s had genetically different steroid metabolism.

These early studies not only involved steroid dosages that are no longer in use but they were not designed to assess the effects of o.c.s on premenstrual changes. Rather, their primary purpose was to assess contraceptive efficacy and the occurrence of side effects in the first few months of contraceptive use. Because of this, no actual assessment of premenstrual changes before and after o.c. use was made and the conclusions that premenstrual changes were abolished or alleviated with o.c. use were based on subjects' spontaneous comments or on very superficial assessment of 'side effects'.

More recent studies have employed a cross-sectional design, i.e. simply comparing women established on o.c.s with non-o.c. users. It is now apparent that such samples are likely to be biased, excluding those women with adverse reactions to o.c.s who will have discontinued their use. A number of studies have found that PMS sufferers are more likely to have experienced such adverse reactions leading to their discontinuing o.c. use in the past than women without premenstrual complaints (e.g. Herzberg *et al.* 1971; Wood *et al.* 1979; Sanders *et al.* 1983; Dennerstein *et al.* 1984). All of these studies have relied on retrospective assessment of reactions to o.c.s; it would be important to study this question in a prospective study.

Very few studies of the effects of o.c.s have used a placebo-controlled design. In the largest study, Cullberg (1972) randomly assigned women to a placebo or one of three combinations of oestrogen and progestagen (the oestrogen dose being the same in each case, the progestagen dose varying). All the women were using other methods of contraception and were told that they were being given a 'mild hormone'. The hormones were taken for two months, and although the number of women involved was impressive ($N = 322$), the methods of assessment were limited and crude. Nevertheless, Cullberg found that women with a previous history of premenstrual irritability showed more adverse reactions to the hormone combinations than to the placebo, particularly the 'oestrogen-dominant' combination. Morris & Udry (1972) studied 51 women, all using other methods of contraception, who took a monophasic o.c., a sequential o.c. (which was later withdrawn from the market) or a placebo for three months. Daily ratings of whether the women felt 'the same', 'better' or 'worse' than usual were made, and little difference was found between the three regimes.

Bancroft *et al.* (1987*a*) randomly assigned women, who wanted to start on oral contraception, to either a monophasic or triphasic preparation (both containing ethinyl oestradiol and levonorgestrel) and monitored them with daily ratings over the first two cycles of use. Among the women who did not normally experience premenstrual mood changes, they found no difference in the effects of the two preparations, but among those who usually experienced negative mood premenstrually, the triphasic preparation was associated with more negative mood change, starting relatively early in the o.c. cycle.

A number of recent studies have used retrospective ratings to compare the pattern and severity of perimenstrual symptoms in o.c. users and non-users. Warner & Bancroft (1988) analysed the peaks and troughs of well being in the cycles of 359 monophasic o.c. users, 283 triphasic users and 3252 women not using steroidal contraception. In general the o.c. users reported less peaks of well being at any stage of the cycle, and less premenstrual troughs, but the monophasic users were more likely to report troughs of well being during the menstrual phase.

Graham & Sherwin (1987) compared 101 o.c. users and 149 non-users by means of the Premenstrual Assessment Form (Halbreich *et al.* 1982). They found the type and number of premenstrual symptoms to be similar in the two groups, but the o.c. users had lower severity scores on several symptoms and a tendency for their symptoms to start closer to the onset of menstrual bleeding than the non-users. The method of assessment used in this study did not indicate the extent to which symptoms were experienced during the menstrual phase.

Bancroft & Rennie (1993) compared 171 monophasic o.c. users, 105 triphasic users and 276 non-o.c. controls, all of whom regarded themselves as PMS sufferers. These subjects were selected from the larger group reported earlier (Warner & Bancroft, 1988) and were matched for age, marital status and parity. hence this study was not concerned with whether o.c. users were more or less likely to experience premenstrual symptoms, but rather to compare the type and pattern of symptoms among those who *were* experiencing cyclical changes. Individual symptoms were rated on a six-point severity scale for the most recent premenstrual week, menstrual days and post-menstrual week. Few differences were found between the two groups except that o.c. users reported much less pain, both menstrually and premenstrually, and less premenstrual breast tenderness. In view of the strong association between period pain and depressive mood found in another study using the same methods of assessment (Bancroft *et al.* 1993 *a*), the two groups were further matched for the severity of menstrual pain. When this was done it was found that the o.c. users, while similar to the non-users in the severity of negative mood during the premenstrual week, showed less improvement in negative mood during the menstrual phase and to some extent, during the postmenstrual week as well. Thus, when the confounding effect of pain was controlled, the o.c. users either had more prolonged perimenstrual negative mood changes or their negative mood change started later in the premenstrual week (as had been found by Graham & Sherwin (1987)) and hence remitted later. The distinction between these two explanations could not be made because of the nature of the retrospective ratings used.

A few studies have compared o.c. users and non-users with daily ratings. Marriot & Faragher (1986) compared 34 o.c. users and 31 non-users over 32 days and found no differences between the groups. Walker & Bancroft (1990) compared 30 triphasic, 35 monophasic and 57 non-steroidal contraceptors over two cycles. All of the subjects had answered 'yes' or 'maybe' to the question 'Do you suffer from PMS?' and the three groups were matched for age and parity. The most striking finding in this study was the similarity

of the three groups, regardless of the method of analysing their daily reports. Two symptoms showed differences; breast tenderness occurred to a similar extent in the controls and triphasic users, but substantially less in the monophasic users; the monophasic group were more likely to show low mood during the menstrual phase, consistent with the earlier findings based on retrospective ratings (Warner & Bancroft, 1988).

The differences in breast tenderness were attributed by Walker & Bancroft (1990) to a greater tendency for monophasic o.c.s than triphasics to completely suppress follicular development, a difference that had been reported previously (Kuhl *et al.* 1985). The suggestion was that the breast changes depended on some degree of follicular development whether or not ovulation followed. To pursue this possibility, McNeill (1992) compared 10 monophasic and 10 triphasic o.c. users, monitoring their cycles with both daily ratings of symptoms and daily early morning urine samples to allow measurement of oestrone glucuronide. Against expectation, she found no difference between the two o.c. groups in the extent to which follicular development occurred, and no association between follicular development and mood changes, although there was an association with breast tenderness. It is important to emphasize that the degree of follicular development involved in this study resulted in endogenous oestrogen levels which were substantially lower than those occurring during normal ovarian cycles. But as McNeill found in a second study (McNeill, 1992), the occasional woman does show much higher levels of oestrogen during o.c. cycles, presumably due to multiple follicular development.

Only one placebo-controlled study has evaluated the effects of o.c.s as a treatment for PMS. Graham & Sherwin (1992) assessed 82 women seeking treatment for PMS with daily ratings before treatment, and then randomly allocated them to either a triphasic o.c. (*Synphasic*, Syntex) or placebo for three months, continuing daily ratings of symptoms throughout. Although more women dropped out of treatment on the active o.c. than on placebo (17:5), of those who completed treatment, significant improvement in mood symptoms were reported by both the o.c. and the placebo groups. The only symptoms to show significantly greater improvement with

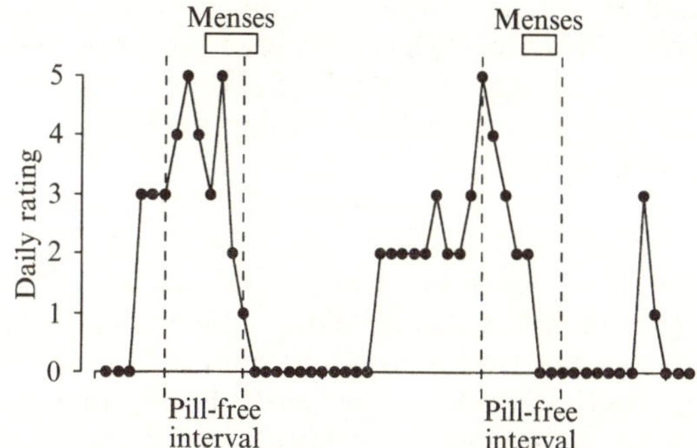



FIG. 2. Daily ratings of depression in a woman taking a combined oral contraceptive. In each of the two o.c. cycles, depressive mood starts before the pill-free interval, showing that the mood change is not simply a result of steroid withdrawal. (From McNeill, 1992.)

the o.c. than with placebo were breast tenderness and bloating. Interestingly, the o.c. group showed a significant worsening of sexual interest during the menstrual and postmenstrual phases of the cycle, an effect which did not occur in the placebo group.

While the evidence of the effects of o.c.s is now building up, the picture remains somewhat confused. A proportion of women, of unknown size, do appear to show adverse mood reactions to o.c. use and as a consequence are likely to discontinue their use at an early stage (Bancroft & Sartorius, 1990). A number of studies have suggested that breast tenderness may be less evident in women taking o.c.s (Walker & Bancroft, 1990; Graham & Sherwin, 1992; Bancroft & Rennie, 1993). There is some evidence that during o.c. cycles, particularly of the combined monophasic variety, the pattern of mood change is slightly altered perhaps due to a withdrawal effect lowering mood during the pill-free interval. However, this effect does not appear to be marked. Furthermore, it is not unusual to find women complaining of PMS while taking monophasic o.c.s, in whom daily monitoring clearly shows the onset of symptoms during the pill-taking phase of the cycle and before the pill free interval. An example of this is shown in Fig. 2.

The most consistent beneficial effect of o.c.s on perimenstrual symptoms involve physical changes, in particular period-type pain. In so far as menstrual pain may aggravate perimenstrual mood, o.c.s may have other indirect beneficial effects. Otherwise o.c.s appear to be no better

than placebo in improving premenstrual mood changes.

The evidence that o.c.s have an adverse though subtle effect on sexuality should be investigated further.

In general, it is difficult to reconcile these relatively subtle differences between the cyclical symptoms occurring with o.c.s and during natural ovarian cycles, with a fundamental role for ovulation or corpus luteum activity in the causation of PMS. Although it can be stated that an o.c. regime does represent a cyclical hormonal regime, the endocrine similarities with the normal ovarian cycle are exceedingly crude, even with the triphasic form of o.c. Further careful research to pursue the subtle differences of symptom patterns that have been observed is indicated.

## D. Other methods of altering the ovarian cycle

### (i) Oestrogen implants and patches

Comparable to oral contraception is the administration of oestrogen, as widely used for hormone replacement following oophorectomy or the menopause. Oestrogen implants or transdermal patches have also been used for the treatment of PMS. Magos *et al.* (1984), in an uncontrolled study, reported success with 50 mg oestradiol implants at 6 monthly intervals. They went on to evaluate this treatment in a placebo-controlled, parallel design study in which 33 women received 100 mg oestradiol implants plus 5 mg oral norethisterone for 7 days each month, and 35 women received placebo implants and placebo tablets (Magos *et al.* 1986*b*). There was a remarkably high placebo response, with 94% of the placebo group showing improvement during the first 2 months. However, the placebo response waned whereas the response to active implants did not. The long-term effects of the considerable amount of oestradiol that is administered to young cycling women with such treatment are not known. One puzzling feature of this report is the apparent lack of any adverse reaction to the intermittent progestagen, particularly as these same workers published a study in the same year (Magos *et al.* 1986*a*), showing a convincing adverse effect of the same progestagen used in the same way for post-menopausal women receiving oestradiol implants (see below). Perhaps there were more disadvantages from the progestagens than were admitted in this report. Three years later this group writes that the use of intermittent progestagens to protect the endometrium 'may produce intolerable cyclical symptoms: up to 10 % of patients treated long-term by oestradiol implants require hysterectomy' (Watson *et al.* 1989).

Watson *et al.* (1989) evaluated the effects of oestradiol transcutaneous patches in a placebo-controlled study. They claimed 'to have shown the effectiveness of percutaneous patches in the treatment of premenstrual syndrome', but their study is curiously flawed. Forty women, shown to have cyclical symptoms, were given 3 months of oestradiol patches and 3 months of placebo patches. The order was balanced, one group of 20 women having the active patches first, another group of 20, the placebo first. Progestagen (5 mg norethisterone for 7 days per month) was given to protect the endometrium and to regulate bleeding. However, the intermittent progestagen was given with *both* the active and the placebo patches. Results showed an improvement in most symptoms over the first 3 months in both groups, with placebo patches being as effective as the active treatment. When subjects crossed over at 3 months, those changing from active treatment to placebo lost their improvement, while those changing from placebo to active continued to improve. The key problem with this study is that the placebo treatment was not simple placebo, but involved intermittent progestagens which have been shown by this group (Magos *et al.* 1986*c*) and others (Hammarbäck *et al.* 1985; Sherwin, 1991) to produce symptoms similar to PMS. We will consider this effect of progestagens later. While this study is of interest, the conclusiveness of the results, as presented by the authors, must be questioned. It is also noteworthy that they used a high dose of oestradiol patch (i.e. 200 $\mu$g every 3 days) which is likely to produce sustained high levels of circulating oestradiol, and is four times greater than the usual dose for hormone replacement. This dose had been shown to suppress ovulation in a previous study (Watson *et al.* 1988), but the effectiveness, or otherwise, of lower doses in suppressing ovulation was not reported.

### (*ii*) *Danazol*

This synthetic steroid is a derivative of 17-$\alpha$-ethinyl testosterone, which is widely assumed to have antigonadotrophic as well as weak androgenic properties. It has been used for more than 25 years for the treatment of endometriosis. In sufficient dosage it blocks ovulation and results in amenorrhoea.

Its use in the treatment of PMS was first reported by Day (1979) who concluded that it may be of value in intractable cases, but with higher doses (400 mg daily and above) side effects were troublesome. Mansel *et al.* (1982) reported a placebo-controlled study of danazol in the treatment of cyclical breast pain, a common symptom of PMS, although no information was given as to whether the women in the study suffered from other cyclical symptoms, or how such symptoms responded to this treatment. Danazol was effective, in a dose-related manner, in relieving breast pain, although the higher dose used (400 mg daily) was associated with more severe side effects. No evidence was reported of the effects of treatment on ovulation or menstrual bleeding.

Only two placebo-controlled studies of the treatment of PMS with danazol have been reported, both with design problems. Watts *et al.* (1987) used a parallel group design to compare 100, 200 and 400 mg daily of danazol with placebo. The numbers were too small for this type of design (10 in each group) and there were important group differences in the severity of symptoms before treatment which served to confound treatment effects. They nevertheless concluded that danazol was effective in reducing breast pain, lethargy, anxiety and increased appetite, but no more effective than placebo for the other symptoms. Anovulation was invariable with the 400 mg dosage, and less likely with the 200 mg. These authors recommended, on somewhat uncertain grounds, that 200 mg was the optimum dose and commented that while symptom relief did not depend on suppression of menstrual bleeding, it *might* be associated with anovulation.

Sarno *et al.* (1987), in a placebo-controlled cross-over study of 14 women with PMS, used danazol in an unusual manner; 200 mg daily (or placebo) was taken 'only from the onset of symptoms until the onset of menses'. A significant superiority of danazol over placebo was found, although such benefit was not found to predominate for any specific type of symptom (including breast tenderness). As to be expected with such a regime, all women continued to ovulate and cycle length and menstrual bleeding were unaffected.

Thus, whereas danazol clearly can be beneficial in relieving symptoms of PMS, and clinical experience supports this, the best controlled evidence of its efficacy that we currently have involves a treatment regime which clearly does not block ovulation or alter menstrual bleeding. The description of danazol as predominantly an antigonadotrophic agent is probably a misleading oversimplification. Barbieri & Ryan (1981) summarized its effects as follows: (a) it prevents the mid-cycle surge of LH and FSH; (b) binds to androgen, progesterone and glucocorticoid, but not oestradiol receptors; (c) binds to sex hormone binding globulin (SHBG) and corticosteroid binding globulin; (d) inhibits multiple enzymes of steroidogenesis; (e) increases the metabolic clearance rate of progesterone; and (f) has hormonally active metabolites. Given this complexity of action, the somewhat inconsistent findings reported above are less surprising. But this also means that the effects of danazol are relatively unhelpful in our attempts to understand the endocrine determinants of PMS.

### (iii) LHRH analogues

A powerful method of blocking ovulation without involvement of exogenous steroids arrived with the introduction of LHRH agonists. These initially overstimulate the pituitary to release gonadotrophins leading to down-regulation of pituitary receptors and subsequent inhibition of gonadotrophin release.

The first published report of their use in the treatment of PMS came from Muse *et al.* (1984). Only 8 women were involved, in a single-blind, placebo-controlled cross-over study, using daily subcutaneous self-injections of either 50 $\mu$g of the agonist, supplied by the Salk Institute, or of placebo, each for 3 months. During the first month, when the agonist was producing increased levels of gonadotrophins and a disorganized hormonal picture, the two treatments were not clearly different, although it appears from the data presented that the physical symptoms were already less with the agonist than with the placebo during this first phase. By the second and third months the differences were clear cut, with both physical and emotional symptoms alleviated during agonist cycles. Not only was ovulation blocked, there was also

effective suppression of ovarian steroid production with plasma oestradiol stabilizing at $19 \pm 15$ pg/ml during the second and third months.

These results were striking although no information was given about the degree of placebo response and also why only 8 out of 50 possible women were chosen for this study. It was apparent that although all women showed cyclical symptoms, (their mean symptom scores for the luteal phase had to be more than twice their mean folicular phase scores), 4 women were experiencing substantial levels of symptoms during the folicular phase. However, this experiment should be seen as assessing the effects of not just anovulation but also ovarian suppression, producing a post-menopausal steroid profile which could only be maintained for a short time. Menstrual bleeding occurred during the first month on agonist but not during the second or third months.

The other placebo-controlled treatment study (Hammarbäck & Bäckström, 1988) differs in one particularly important way. The agonist used (buserelin; Svenska Hoechst AB) was administered by nasal spray, which is a less potent method of administration than subcutaneous injection, and a dose was chosen (400 $\mu$g daily in one single dose) which would block ovulation without interfering with menstrual bleeding or substantially suppressing follicular development and cyclical oestradiol production. This paper is difficult to follow, mainly because of an unusual method of statistical analysis which tends to obscure the size of treatment effects. Clearly there was a substantial placebo effect. Beyond that the additional improvement with the agonist looks, from the graphs published, to be modest as far as the emotional changes were concerned, and certainly less dramatic than that reported in the first study. However, the authors concluded that there was a significant and convincing treatment effect of the agonist, in this case when the principal endocrine effect was anovulation.

The apparently clear-cut results with these two studies are in striking contrast with those obtained by our group (Bancroft *et al.* 1987*b*). We studied long-term buserelin administration (by nasal spray doses ranging from 400 to 800 $\mu$g daily, in divided doses) in 20 women with established PMS. As this was regarded as an initial exploratory study, placebo control was not used systematically, though some interesting observations were made with single-blind placebo interventions. In general, the therapeutic effects were much more varied than apparent in the first two studies. In 10 women benefits were sufficient to lead the women to continue on treatment for periods ranging from 5 to 15 months. But in the other 10 women, treatment produced aggravation of symptoms sufficient to lead to discontinuation after 3 to 11 weeks. These varied effects have been documented more fully in other publications (Bancroft *et al.* 1985, 1987*c*). The symptoms showing deterioration varied from woman to woman, though bloating was most consistent in this respect. Bleeding, with an unpredictable and irregular pattern, continued for most women, although 6 eventually became amenorrhoeic after 1 to 7 months of treatment. Noteworthy was the occurrence of physical symptoms such as breast tenderness or bloating in the few days before any menstrual bleed, albeit of lesser severity than occurred pre-treatment. Mood changes showed less temporal linkage to the menstrual bleeding as time went on. These findings suggested that, whereas mood changes became 'detached' from menstrual bleeding by the regime, physical changes continued to show a link in spite of ovulation being blocked in every case. When menstrual bleeding did occur it was normally preceded by a modest rise and fall of oestrogen. Also of interest was the finding that in several women who had stabilized, with ovarian suppression and control of symptoms, the single-blind replacement of the buserelin with placebo resulted in the reappearance of symptoms *before* ovulation had occurred but after some degree of follicular development had taken place.

One suggestion from this study was that the reduction of symptoms was determined not by the absence of ovulation but by the flattening of ovarian steroid production. In one woman the initiation of treatment was followed by a marked worsening of symptoms accompanied by a substantial increase in her urinary oestrogen excretion, suggestive of marked follicular development. This settled and she became asymptomatic. It was tempting to conclude that this early flare-up was the result of the treatment induced oestrogen rise. However, the probability that this explanation is an oversimplification was indicated by her response to administration

later of exogenous oestrogens when no increase in symptoms ensued.

Concerned with the long-term consequences of ovarian suppression by LHRH agonists, Mortola *et al.* (1991) examined the effects of combining agonist induced ovarian suppression with cyclical steroid replacement. Eight women with demonstrable PMS started on an LHRH agonist (histrelin, Ortho; 100 $\mu$g s.c. daily) used alone for 2 months. This resulted in a substantial reduction in premenstrual symptoms. For the next 4 months four separate regimes were administered in double blind fashion, placebo, oestrogen alone for 25 days, progestagen (medroxyprogesterone acetate 10 mg daily) alone for 10 days, and a combination of the oestrogen and progestagen, each for 1 month.

The authors concluded that a relapse of symptoms occurred with three of the regimes (oestrogen alone, progestagen alone, and placebo), but significant improvement was maintained by the combined regime. On the face of it, these results appear to conflict with other studies demonstrating an adverse effect of progestagen when added to oestrogen replacement in post-menopausal women (see below; Hammarbäck *et al.* 1985; Magos *et al.* 1986*c*; Sherwin, 1991). However, this report can be criticized on several grounds. First when using a regime which disrupts bleeding patterns, it is a complex issue to compare premenstrual symptoms pre-treatment and post-treatment (see Bancroft *et al.* 1987*b*). No details of bleeding patterns after the onset of agonist were given, though it is likely that amenorrhoea would have become established before long. It is not, however, acceptable to compare the last 4 premenstrual days pre-treatment, with the last 4 days of the calendar month during treatment, as was done in this paper. It is important to establish with such treatment that overall the woman is better off, and even if she is not getting the marked premenstrual downswings, that she is not feeling generally worse for the rest of the time. Also the comparison of 4 treatments, of one month duration each, in only 8 subjects is unrealistic. No adequate control for order can be achieved (24 subjects would be required for this purpose) not to mention analysis of carry over effects, which are likely to be important in short treatments of this kind. The statistical analysis was not clearly presented. While this study is interesting, we should be cautious before accepting their conclusion that a combined hormone replacement regime is superior to either oestrogen alone, progestagen alone or placebo. Further studies of this kind, with a more appropriate design, are required.

### (*iv*) *Oophorectomy*

If LHRH agonists provide a form of 'medical oophorectomy', the surgical removal of the ovaries, combined with hysterectomy and oestrogen replacement, provides a more drastic but conclusive method of eliminating ovarian activity. Casper & Hearn (1990) reported on 14 women treated in this way: 'Psychological measures 6 months after operation showed dramatic improvement in mood, general affect, well being, life satisfaction and overall quality of life'. Casson *et al.* (1990) reported a further 14 women treated in a similar way with comparable results. These two studies both involved treatment with danazol prior to surgery. In the first, however, this was given for the 3 months immediately preceding surgery. In the second study, danazol was continued, with increasing dosage until amenorrhoea was established, and then maintained on that dosage for several months. The treatment was then stopped and surgical treatment offered as an option if severe PMS returned. This raises the interesting question of whether women who do not respond favourably to danazol would show the same benefits of ovariectomy. Casson *et al.* (1990) commented that menstrual symptoms (e.g. dysmenorrhoea or menorrhagia) were not a feature of the women they treated. Casper & Hearn (1990) did not comment on this important point.

### (*v*) *Effects of intermittent progestagens*

Perhaps the greatest paradox in the field of PMS concerns the role of progesterone. Dalton (1984), one of the earliest proponents of the concept of PMS, has continued to insist that progesterone, administered daily, preferably by injection or failing that by suppository, is a highly effective treatment for 'true' PMS. One of the favoured early aetiological theories was that PMS resulted from a relative deficiency of progesterone, or a relatively high oestradiol/progesterone ratio. The weight of hormonal evidence, which has been reviewed previously

(e.g. Bancroft & Bäckström, 1985) is now against such explanations, and with one unconvincing exception (Dennerstein *et al.* 1985), the placebo controlled treatment outcome studies of natural progesterone, given in the second half of the cycle, have failed to show any superiority over placebo (Sampson, 1979; Van der Meer *et al.* 1983; Maddocks *et al.* 1986). Sampson (1979) found some evidence that adverse reactions were more likely with 800 mg than 400 mg daily. Controlled studies with synthetic progestagens, such as dydrogesterone (Sampson *et al.* 1988; Williams *et al.* 1983), norethisterone (Coppen *et al.* 1969; 7·5 mg daily) or medroxyprogesterone acetate (MPA) (Jordheim, 1972; 7·5 mg daily) have given predominantly negative results, although evidence of a worsening of symptoms has not been prominent. West (1990) compared both MPA (15 mg daily for 21 days) and norethisterone (NET) 15 mg daily for 21 days, with placebo. Apart from an improvement in breast tenderness, the NET was no better than placebo. MPA, on the other hand, did show more general benefits, particularly in those women whose symptoms had previously been confined to the premenstrual phase. Both progestagens blocked ovulation and the NET resulted in greater ovarian suppression than the MPA. But for some unexplained reason the MPA was associated with considerable disruption of the normal bleeding pattern, with frequent breakthrough bleeds, whereas the NET did not alter the bleeding pattern. West, therefore, made the interesting suggestion that the benefits of MPA were related to its disruption of the normal cycle rather than its blocking of ovulation. Four women, two using each progestagen, withdrew from the study because of an aggravation of their premenstrual symptoms. The role of progestagens as treatment for PMS therefore remains confused though not conclusively negative, and any tendency for progestagens to *aggravate* rather than alleviate symptoms seems confined to a small proportion of PMS sufferers.

In contrast to this picture, however, are the interesting observations of the effects of intermittent progestagens when given in combination with oestrogens in hormone replacement of postmenopausal or post-oophorectomized women.

Magos *et al.* (1986*c*) studied 58 post-menopausal hysterectomized women who were receiving subcutaneous oestradiol and testosterone implants. They compared, in double-blind fashion, the effects of norethisterone (2·5 or 5 mg daily for 7 days) with placebo for 7 days. They found widespread adverse effects associated with the progestagen, worse on the higher dosage: 'Symptoms were similar to the typical complaints of the premenstrual syndrome', and they suggested that this combined hormonal regime provided a 'model for the premenstrual syndrome'. Hammarbäck *et al.* (1985) compared cyclical oestradiol (administered transdermally) on its own with an oestrogen/progestagen combination, giving Lynestrenol 5 mg daily during the last 11 days of the oestrogen cycle. There was no placebo control in this study, but similar adverse effects of the progestagen were observed, leading these authors to suggest that 'progestagens are involved in the provocation of cyclical symptom changes seen in the premenstrual syndrome'. One important difference between these two studies is that in one, using implants, the oestrogen levels should have been stable, whereas in the other the oestradiol was given in a cyclical fashion. The similarity of the findings in the two studies therefore indicates that the adverse reaction is not simply a matter of experiencing an intermittent steroid regime. In some way the progestagen was specifically responsible.

A further careful study was reported by Sherwin (1991). Forty-eight naturally menopausal women were randomly assigned to one of four cyclical treatment regimes. Two doses of conjugated equine-oestrogen (CEE) were used (0·625 mg and 1·25 mg daily from days 1 to 25) and combined with either medroxyprogesterone acetate (MPA; 5 mg daily from days 15 to 25) or placebo for the same time period. Once again the progestagen was associated with an increase in psychological symptoms, an effect that was less noticeable when combined with the higher oestrogen dose.

This progestagen effect, which bedevils much of hormone replacement therapy for postmenopausal women, is therefore of considerable theoretical interest, and the apparent conflict with the PMS treatment data remains puzzling. It is of course possible that the effects of intermittent progestagens are different in a woman with an already established post-menopausal endocrine status, with its altered CNS pattern of response to steroid feedback. In addition, it is important to remember that not only may synthetic progestagens differ from natural progesterone in this respect (not only directly but also via differences in bioactive metabolites) there may also be important differences between the varieties of synthetic progestagens. Certainly, more research on these adverse effects of progestagens is needed.

## E. Does the cyclical pattern represent an entrained rhythm in the brain?

Clinical experience gives examples of how apparently clear cyclical patterns of symptoms can show variable temporal relationship to menstruation, particular when menstrual bleeding is somewhat irregular. In an earlier review (Bancroft & Bäckstrom, 1985) we postulated that the mood changes of PMS are centrally determined and that the timing of their cyclicity results from the interaction between some central regulator and ovarian feedback.

In an interesting study, Schmidt *et al.* (1991) interfered with the normal ovarian cycle in a double-blind fashion. In one experimental condition, established PMS sufferers were given an antiprogestagen, mifepristone, on the 7th day after the LH surge. This induced luteolysis and menstrual bleeding within 2 to 3 days. In a second condition, the mifepristone was combined with HCG, with the result that early menstrual bleeding was induced but luteal function was maintained, with a subsequent further bleed at the usual time. In the third condition, placebo alone was given. In spite of these manipulations of both luteal function and menstrual bleeding, the timing and extent of premenstrual symptoms continued in a similar fashion in the three groups. These authors offered two explanations for these findings: (a) that the process of premenstrual change was triggered earlier in the cycle, before the intervention occurred and continued to run its course unaffected – this would be consistent with the idea that ovulation is the key event; (b) that premenstrual symptoms are part of a cyclic mood disturbance that is synchronized with the menstrual cycle but not caused by it. The effect of the intervention would be to desynchronize the two phenomena in a manner analogous to 'jet lag' in the traveller.

This second possibility was investigated further by McNeill (1992) who used the combined oral contraceptive (Marvelon, Organon) as a means of manipulating the hormonal cycle. Women established on o.c.s were randomly assigned to one of two double-blind regimes. In each case, the subject took a pill every day; in one regime this gave her 21 days of active pill and 7 days of placebo, i.e. a normal o.c. cycle. In the other regime an active pill was taken continuously for 4 to 5 months. In the 16 women who completed the continuous regime, 10 continued to show cyclical patterns of at least one type of symptom in spite of suppressed ovarian activity and no menstrual bleeding. The symptoms which showed this 'free-running rhythm' most convincingly were physical symptoms such as bloating or breast tenderness. But three women showed convincing examples of mood changes, as well as physical symptoms, 'free running' in this way.

These findings indicate that, at least in some women, a well established cyclical pattern will continue to 'free run' in the presence of a suppressed or stable hormonal milieu, suggesting an endogenous or at least entrained rhythm in the central nervous system. How long such 'free running' might continue is not clear, but appears to be at least 3 or 4 months. It is therefore perhaps surprising that no clear examples of such 'free running' have been reported in the studies of ovarian suppression with LHRH analogues. This may be because the initial stimulating effect of the agonist, which might include direct effects on the CNS, could serve to disrupt the pattern. Obviously more research into this interesting and crucial possibility is warranted. It is also worth considering the possible relevance of the high number of ovulatory cycles that the modern woman experiences (MacDonald *et al.* 1991) and whether this serves to reinforce and entrain CNS rhythms over a period of time. In a previous study, we found some association between the likelihood of reporting PMS and the duration of an uninterrupted span of natural cycles (Warner & Bancroft, 1990).

## F. Aetiological conclusions so far

The notion that PMS depends on ovulation and luteal activity and that effective treatment is a function of ovulation suppression appears increasingly to be an over-simplification of the evidence. On the one hand, there is convincing evidence that disruption of the normal ovarian cycle *may* result in substantial reduction of cyclical symptoms; on the other hand, there is evidence, so far limited, that in some sense the cyclicity of symptoms represents some rhythm in the brain, entrained or reinforced by a cyclical hormonal regime, which may be serving little function beyond that of a time keeper. The possibility that ovulation acts as a trigger for such a time-keeping process has been suggested (Schmidt *et al.* 1991), but it would appear that the time keeping can be achieved equally well by an o.c. cycle in which no more than trivial follicular development occurs, and certainly no ovulation. The idea that what is required for effective treatment is a stable hormonal state deserves further consideration. Maybe in such circumstances any entrained rhythm will sooner or later become extinguished. But this notion of stability, at least in women with intact uteri, is difficult to study because of the need to protect the endometrium from unopposed oestrogen. The notion of stability is also not straightforward. In McNeill's (1992) study, in which an oestrogen–progestagen combination was taken continuously for several months, there was, apart from the evidence of 'free running' rhythms in some women, also a tendency for breakthrough bleeding to occur sooner or later. This happened in the majority of women, but was apparently unassociated with any significant variation in endogenous steroid levels. The cause of such bleeding remains obscure, but it would appear that a 'stable' state is difficult to achieve with this form of exogenous hormone administration.

The intriguing paradox regarding progestagens remains. Why is there such convincing evidence of the 'simulation' of PMS by intermittent progestagens, when so many clinicians rely on intermittent progestagens as a form of treatment? It is one thing to criticize such regimes as being no better than placebo, but it is another to suggest that they predictably recreate or aggravate the PMS pattern.

At this stage of the analysis we can perhaps claim less naivety than was prominent a few years ago. There is less expectation that we will find the answer in some abnormality of the ovarian cycle, or in abnormal levels of some key factor during the late luteal phase. But the questions still outweigh the answers, and the mystery has not lessened.

## IV. A PARADIGM SHIFT – THE THREE-FACTOR MODEL

Two recent studies from the author's group have provoked ideas which, while not particularly new or surprising, are, we believe, helpful in reformulating the complex situation that confronts us in this review.

The first study set out to establish whether biological markers which have been associated with depressive illness are present in women experiencing perimenstrual depression; in other words, do these two types of depressive mood experience have any underlying neurobiological mechanisms in common? The markers looked at were the neuroendocrine responses to intravenous (i.v.) L-tryptophan, the precursor of serotonin. Normally a challenge of this kind results in increased levels of plasma prolactin and growth hormone. These responses have been shown to be blunted in depressive illness (see below). This neuroendocrine challenge test was therefore carried out twice, once in the late luteal 'premenstrual' phase and again in the mid-follicular 'postmenstrual' phase. Two groups of women were compared, one showing a premenstrual pattern of depression, the other showing no depressive mood changes at the time of the tests (Bancroft *et al.* 1991). We found premenstrual blunting of prolactin response *in both groups of women*. In contrast, we found blunting of the GH and cortisol response in the women with premenstrual depression, *but in both phases of the cycle*. The prolactin response to tryptophan is probably mediated by serotonin; the mediation of the GH and cortisol responses is less clear. We postulated that the blunted prolactin response was reflecting an alteration of brain serotonergic activity that normally occurs at this stage of the cycle but which is clearly not sufficient itself to lead to mood change – we referred to this as a '*timing factor*'. In contrast, blunting of GH and cortisol responses was not apparently related to the ovarian cycle, as in both cases it was present at both phases of the cycle tested. (The possible mediation of these different responses will be considered in more detail later.) We therefore postulated that these altered responses reflected some ongoing *vulnerability* of the women, not itself determined by the hormonal cycle but which, when combined with the late luteal 'timing factor', led to mood change at that particular phase (i.e. the premenstrual phase) of the cycle.

This is a 'paradigm shift', because whereas previously aetiological research had been dominated by the search for 'abnormalities' of the ovarian cycle in women with PMS, here were discriminatory differences between women with and without premenstrual mood change which were not related to the phase of the ovarian cycle. Whether such differences are 'state' or 'trait' abnormalities is not yet possible to say, but what this evidence suggested is that a combination of (i) a relatively normal ovarian cycle-related phenomenon, present in the majority of women, and (ii) some other non-cycle related characteristic, results in the complaints that women present as 'premenstrual syndrome'. This was not the first time that this type of result had been reported in neurobiological studies and we will be considering other comparable findings below. Rubinow & Schmidt (1992) reacted to this type of evidence, in which the distinguishing features of the PMS sufferer appear to be independent of cycle phase, by proposing their 'state' model of PMS. This makes use of the 'state' concept propounded by Wolff (1987), among others, in which the normal human condition consists of a variety of highly organized experiential or behavioural states, reflecting coherent beliefs, perceptions, affects as well as neurobiological characteristics, which determine how the individual interacts with her environment. Thus, Rubinow & Schmidt (1992) conclude 'In this framework, PMS can be seen as a disorder characterised by a menstrual cycle-linked transition into a particular experiential state that is usually (although not exclusively) characterised by dysphoria or irritability.... the menstrual cycle facilitates the state change but does not produce the symptoms directly' (p. 51).

The second study from our group was of a very different kind but produced findings which complemented those of the first. It derived from our clinical concern that many women seeking help for so-called 'PMS' do not fit into the usual criteria and yet present problems which appear related to the menstrual cycle in some way and which involve levels of distress that warrant clinical help. We, therefore, set out to compare and contrast women seeking help for menstrual cycle related problems, but who presented their problems as either PMS, menorrhagia or dysmenorrhoea. To what extent is there symptom overlap in these three clinical groups? More important, to what extent may problems with menstruation influence the pre- or peri-menstrual pattern of mood change experienced? Remarkably little attention has been paid to the inter-relationship between these three common gynaecological complaints. Yet when attention has been paid, the evidence of an important inter-relationship is apparent. In particular, dysmenorrhoea and PMS have been linked by several studies (see below).

The association with menorrhagia has been much less studied. But there is a growing belief, although little evidence to support it, that as the majority of women complaining of heavy periods can be shown to have clinically acceptable levels of blood loss, this complaint is in many cases either the somatization of an emotional problem or, at best, a consequence of inappropriate expectations about normal menstruation.

In this recent study (Bancroft *et al.* 1993 *a, b*) three groups of gynaecological clinic attenders were assessed, 101 with the principal complaint of menorrhagia, 104 complaining of premenstrual syndrome and 56 of dysmenorrhoea. A comparison group of 105 women, who had not sought help for any of these three complaints in the previous two years, was recruited from general practice. The assessment of perimenstrual symptoms was based on retrospective ratings of the premenstrual week, the menstrual days and the postmenstrual week of the last menstrual period. Hence the evidence has to be regarded as crude.

First, there was a considerable overlap in our three patient groups. In particular, heavy periods were commonly reported by women in the PMS and dysmenorrhoea groups. Pain was also commonly reported by the PMS and menorrhagia groups, and interestingly, among the dysmenorrhoea complainers, period-type pain most commonly started during the premenstrual phase. In general, women with either severe pain or heavy periods were more likely to report depression, both premenstrually as well as menstrually. There was, therefore, evidence that

menstrual problems did influence the pattern of premenstrual symptoms including mood change.

Two symptoms looked particularly interesting: food craving and clumsiness. Both were more severe in those women who sought help for premenstrual changes than in those who reported such changes but did not seek help for them. Both were particularly marked premenstrually and neither was affected by the menstrual problems of pain or heavy bleeding.

We also examined the relationship between the severity and timing of perimenstrual symptoms and two other non-cycle related factors; 'neuroticism', as measured by the Eysenck Personality Inventory (EPI), and previous history of depressive illness.

'Neuroticism' (N) is an aspect of personality which reflects an increased tendency to suffer common mental health problems such as depressive illness, and also a tendency to seek professional help for such problems (Goldberg & Huxley, 1991). The severity of each of the perimenstrual mood symptoms was highly correlated with N, whereas correlations with other symptoms such as breast tenderness, clumsiness or food craving were low. The associations between symptom patterns and past history of depression is discussed below.

With the results of both this study and L-tryptophan challenge study in mind, we postulated a 'three factor model' to account for the complexities of menstrual cycle-related complaints.

### Factor 1 – the 'timing factor'

This is assumed (*a*) to involve the effects of the hormonal cycle on the brain, possibly mediated by varying levels of neurotransmitter activity; and (*b*) to underlie the mild changes that many women experience premenstrually, but which are usually not sufficiently marked or severe to cause problems or to lead to help-seeking. A 'neutral' label was chosen for this factor to avoid confusion with the pre-existing 'social constructs' that pervade this field.

### Factor 2 – the 'menstruation factor'

This is assumed to involve processes leading up to and during menstruation. Prostaglandins are obvious candidates as mediating factors; during the secretory phase of the cycle these increase in amount in the circulation, as well as in the endometrium. Such changes could be associated not only with increased sensitivity to pain but also with fatigue and negative mood.

## Factor 3 – the 'vulnerability' factor

This involves characteristics of the woman, such as neuroticism or a propensity to depressive illness, which are not directly related to the ovarian cycle, but which may influence how a woman reacts to or copes with menstrual cycle-related changes.

This model represents a 'paradigm shift', which is parallel to that of the 'state' model of Rubinow & Schmidt but, we believe, has greater heuristic value. In particular, it provides us with a different framework for considering research evidence of aetiological relevance. For the remainder of this review, therefore, we will use this framework to consider and re-appraise the evidence. The aim is as much to re-organize the research agenda for the future as to provide answers at present. It is hoped to convince the reader that, by using this framework, the crucial questions and hence the relevant research become more easily identified.

## V. THE ROLE OF THE OVARIAN CYCLE AND THE 'TIMING FACTOR'

If the ovarian cycle induces changes in women's subjective state as a result of its hormonal profile, we should expect to find such changes in a substantial proportion of women, even if they are hardly noticeable or not problematical. Variability of such experiences due to variations in the hormonal profile itself is not likely to be important. The occurrence of short luteal phases or deficient luteal function, as well as anovulation, may contribute to the variability, but such variations are relatively uncommon. Differences between women may reflect genetic or constitutional differences in how they react to hormonal change. Such differences may also be amplified, or even determined by women's varying expectations and attitudes to menstruation.

The term 'timing factor' has been chosen both because of its 'neutrality' and because it implies that any such effect of the ovarian cycle is going to be apparent at a certain stage in the temporal sequence. We will review the evidence for influence of the ovarian cycle on women's subjective experience by first considering various types of subjective experience: mood change, cognitive function, motor co-ordination, appetite, and physical changes such as bloating or breast tenderness. We will then consider the evidence for cyclical variation in CNS activity in terms of either CNS responsiveness or neurotransmitter function.

## A. Mood change

The few studies that have looked at positive changes through the cycle have consistently shown an increase in well-being through the follicular phase, reaching a peak around mid-cycle and declining in the late luteal phase. Sanders *et al.* (1983) compared three groups of women with daily ratings of mood and well-being through the cycle. One group was of women presenting at a clinic complaining of PMS. The other two groups were from volunteers, half of whom regarded themselves as PMS sufferers, the other half reporting no predictable changes in well-being during their cycles. The pattern of well-being in the three groups is shown in Fig. 3. As to be expected, the variation is most marked in the clinic group. The non-PMS volunteers, however, did show a comparable pattern but this was weak and did not reach statistical significance.

A large number of studies have investigated negative mood changes through the cycle in non-clinic women (Asso, 1983). The results, inevitably, have been variable, and the overall impression has varied according to the commentator's standpoint. Thus, Asso (1988) regards the predominant picture as one of increasing negative mood (though not commonly depression) during the premenstrual phase, with 'a small minority of studies which found no significant cyclical variation' (p. 29). Ussher (1992), on the other hand, emphasizes in a recent review 'the growing body of evidence showing no change in mood throughout the menstrual cycle' (page 134). The explanations for this variable picture reflects much of the key controversy in this field. The most crucial issue, which is relevant to the general debate about PMS, is the extent to which cycle-related changes, when reported, are artefacts of the method of enquiry or the consequences of expectation and attribution. There have been four types of study addressing these issues (Graham, 1989) involving assessment of: (a) cultural, stereotypical beliefs about menstru-

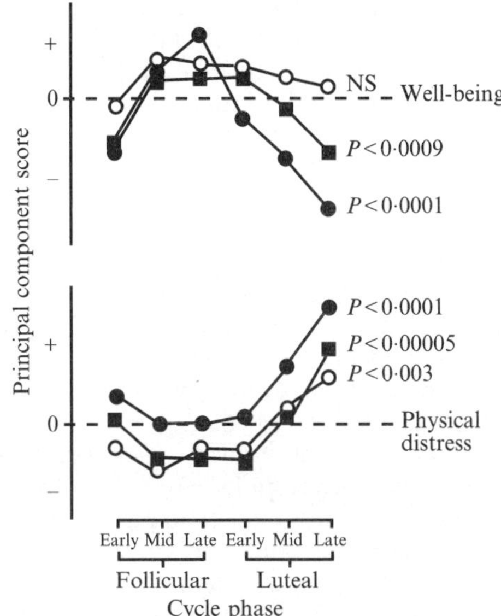



FIG. 3. Principal component scores derived from a variety of daily ratings in three groups of women, averaged for six phases of the hormonal cycle. The first component was labelled 'well-being', the third component 'physical distress'. The three groups were: (i) women attending a PMS clinic (●, Clinic PMS, $N = 19$); (ii) volunteers who regarded themselves as PMS sufferers (■, Non-clinic PMS, $N = 18$); and (iii) volunteers who did not suffer from PMS (○, No PMS, $N = 16$). The $P$ values refer to within-group differences across phases. All three groups showed cycle-related variation in physical distress. Only the two PMS groups showed significant cycle-related variation in well-being, although the 'No PMS' group showed non-significant increases in 'well-being' mid-cycle. (From Sanders *et al.* 1983.)

ation; (b) the effects on self-report of 'focusing' on the menstrual cycle; (c) manipulation of expectancies about whether menstrual cycle changes actually occur; and (d) manipulation of women's beliefs about where they are in their current cycle.

Studies of the first kind have shown that there are cultural beliefs about the effects of the menstrual cycle on women's well being, shared by both women and men (e.g. Parlee, 1974). With the second kind of study, results have varied. Some studies have shown that, when the focus of the study is the menstrual cycle, subjects are more likely to report premenstrual changes (Englander-Golden *et al.* 1978; Parlee, 1982; AuBuchon & Calhoun, 1985). Others have found this not to be the case (Markum, 1976; Van den Akker & Steptoe, 1985) or even the opposite (Rogers & Harding, 1981). Manipulating women's beliefs about whether premenstrual changes occur has been shown to influence symptom reporting (Fradkin & Firestone, 1986;

Olasov & Jackson, 1987). In a much cited study, Ruble (1977) led women to believe that they were either in the premenstrual or intermenstrual phase of the cycle when, in fact, they were not. The women believing themselves to be 'premenstrual' reported more physical symptoms than those believing themselves to be 'intermenstrual'. Interestingly, this effect was not apparent in their reports of negative mood.

It is noteworthy that, without exception, these studies of the effects of expectancy and belief have involved young women with no indication of the proportion who regarded themselves as PMS sufferers. Women seeking help for 'PMS' are likely to be older. In our recent clinic study (Bancroft *et al.* 1993*a*) the average age was 35·9 years (s.d. ±6·4; range 17–48) which is comparable to other clinic based reports (e.g. Keye *et al.* 1986, 34·2 years; Freeman *et al.* 1985, 33 years; Hargrove & Abraham, 1982, 33 years.) Thus, while it is reasonable to conclude that such psychological mechanisms may influence reporting of cycle-related changes in non-complaining volunteers, we have no evidence that such mechanisms are playing a significant part in the reporting of symptoms in those distressed by premenstrual changes.

It is also questionable whether all or even most of the variability in the literature concerning non-clinical subjects can be explained by such 'artefactual' effects. There are other methodological sources of variance (Ussher, 1992). But it is also distinctly possible that there is genuine variability among women in both the extent to which they experience cycle-related changes in well-being, and also the temporal pattern of such changes. A tendency to feel best around mid-cycle and worst premenstrually and menstrually appears to be the commonest pattern, though usually mild and non-problematical. A proportion of women, however, report premenstrual *increases* in well being or energy. In one study 17% of non-clinic subjects were in this category (Halbreich & Endicott, 1982).

## B. Cognitive function

There is now an extensive literature on the relationship between menstrual cycle and cognitive function. Up to 1990, this has been effectively reviewed by Sommer (1992) and her conclusions will be briefly summarized. Studies of abstract thinking, memory, arithmetic, visuospatial ability, and simple speed and time tasks failed to demonstrate any cycle-phase effects. A suggestion of phase effects on verbal performance, with possible premenstrual and menstrual impairment, was probably attributable to speech production and articulation rather than comprehension, and was not a consistent finding.

## C. Psychophysiological reactivity

Measures of cortical arousal and autonomic responsiveness have been studied in relation to the menstrual cycle. This evidence has recently been reviewed by Dye (1992). Arousal and activation of the CNS has principally been investigated by tests of visual acuity or by means of visual information processing tasks. Tests of visual acuity (e.g. light detection threshold) have shown variable results but with a tendency for performance to be optimal around ovulation. Visual information processing, such as shown by the two-flash fusion (TFF) threshold, the interstimulus interval at which the subject reports seeing two successive flashes as one single flash, is obviously influenced by a variety of factors and is not simply a measure of cortical arousal or activation. Most studies, though not all, have reported a higher threshold (i.e. decreased sensitivity) pre- or perimenstrually in 'normal' women. A comparable but subtly different test, the critical flicker fusion threshold (CFFT), was found by Dye (1992) in her own studies to give the *best* performance premenstrually. These somewhat inconsistent results indicate the difficulties in interpreting evidence of this kind.

Tests on autonomic reactivity have mainly involved peripheral changes such as heart rate or electrodermal activity. Once again the results have been variable, but a somewhat more consistent picture has emerged of increased autonomic reactivity during the premenstrual phase (Dye, 1992).

## D. Reactions to stress

Given the likely impact of a woman's current level of adversity on her ability to cope, do women differ in their response to stress at different stages of the cycle? Once again the evidence is inconsistent (Ussher, 1992). Adrenocortical reactivity to experimentally induced stress was shown to be greater during the late premenstrual phase than mid-cycle by Marinari *et al.* (1976), an effect which was not apparent in o.c. users. Ablanalp *et al.* (1977), however, found no difference in cortisol or GH response to mild experimentally induced stress between the menstrual and intermenstrual phases. Collins *et al.* (1985), using time-pressured cognitive tasks as experimental stressors, found no difference in cortisol response in three phases of the cycle (days 5–7, 12–14 and 22–25). They did, however, find that urinary adrenaline and noradrenaline excretion was higher, following the stressor, in the luteal phase.

Hastrup & Light (1984) investigated cardiovascular responses to stress in men and women. The women showed lower heart rate and blood pressure responses to a stressful task during follicular days 7–11 than mid-luteal days 17–21. Interestingly, the men's responses were similar to the higher responses of the women during the luteal phase. Plante & Denney (1984) also used cardiovascular responses to assess the relevance of dysmenorrhoea to perimenstrual responsiveness to stress. No consistent differences in their response to stress were found between women with and without dysmenorrhoea and overall, changes in cardiovascular responses at different stages of the cycle were small.

It is difficult to judge the extent to which these variable results are the consequence of methodological differences, such as timing of tests in the cycle, type of stressor used, response-pattern measured etc., or alternatively reflect individual variability among women in their cycle-related responsiveness. Either or both could be important.

## E. Motor co-ordination

Two studies have shown a cycle-related change in co-ordination of large muscle movement. Zimmerman & Parlee (1973) tested arm-hand steadiness by holding a metal stylus within a hole in a metal plate – the objective being to avoid the stylus touching the plate. They studied 14 young female college students at four stages of the menstrual cycle: menstrual (days 1–4), mid-follicular (days 6–12), early- to mid-luteal (days 17–21) and late luteal or premenstrual (days 23–27). Steadiness was greatest during the early-to mid-luteal phase, with a significant decrement premenstrually. Hudgens *et al.* (1988) used basically the same testing procedure in a larger group of 48 normally cycling women, but also 19 monophasic oral contraceptive users and 58 men, each of the three groups having a mean age of 21 years. They used similar phases of the menstrual cycle as well as repeated testing over more than one cycle. They replicated the findings of Zimmerman & Parlee (1973) in the normally cycling women, but in addition found that these women were in general superior to both the men and the o.c. using women on this task. Their findings suggested that o.c., presumably by flattening out the hormonal cycle, reduced performance on this task during the mid-part of the cycle. They went on in a smaller study to test the effect of attaching the stylus in the barrel of a hand gun, and thus assess steadiness in holding a handgun. The findings were similar. Thus, while this evidence indicates a premenstrual decline in performance, it would appear to be from a level, during most of the cycle, which is generally superior to that found in men! These interesting findings invite comparison with the clumsiness that is often reported by women during the premenstrual phase. In our study discussed above (Bancroft *et al.* 1993*a*) this complaint was apparently unaffected by menstrual problems and only weakly associated with neuroticism raising the possibility that it is linked more directly to the ovarian cycle and our 'timing factor'. However, it is worth considering the possibility that this 'premenstrual clumsiness' is also a decline in performance to a level comparable to that in the average man.

Other more subtle effects, such as in pursuit rotor tracking, preferred tapping rate, and 'psychomotor reminiscence' have also been related to cycle phase, though no consistent picture of premenstrual/menstrual impairment emerged (Sommer, 1992). Clearly, careful analysis of premenstrual complaints of clumsiness, and more cycle-related research on the types of motor co-ordination relevant to such clumsiness, is warranted.

### F. Appetite

In the previously discussed study (Bancroft *et al.* 1993*a*) appetite change, in particular food craving, suggested itself as a potentially useful marker of the 'timing factor'. To what extent does appetite or food craving vary with the menstrual cycle? Many women experience changes in appetite during the cycle, with increased food intake during the luteal phase (Dalvit, 1981; Dalvit-McPhillips, 1983; Pilner & Fleming, 1983; Bowen & Grunberg, 1990). These appetite changes are often characterized by craving for sweet food or chocolate.

Premenstrual food craving is a common complaint of women with 'PMS'. In a study of 5457 women, most of whom regarded themselves as PMS sufferers, 36% reported 'severe' craving for sweet foods around the time of menstruation, 7% reported 'severe' cravings for salty foods and 11% for other types of food (Warner & Bancroft, 1988). In a clinic population of PMS sufferers, 24% complained of sweet-food craving (Hargrove & Abraham, 1982). Changes in taste sensitivity, preference and actual calorific consumption were found to be increased premenstrually in women with PMS (Blundell & Hill, 1989; Wurtman *et al.* 1989).

Although Both-Orthman *et al.* (1988) found premenstrual craving to be more severe in women with premenstrual depression than in controls, it has been clearly demonstrated in women without any mood change (Cohen *et al.* 1987; Bancroft *et al.* 1988), and when the two phenomena do co-exist, they appear to be relatively independent of each other (Cohen *et al.* 1987; Bancroft *et al.* 1988; Schechter *et al.* 1989). It is nevertheless possible that both share some underlying aetiological factor, without such a factor being sufficient for either to be manifested. A likely candidate for this common factor is an alteration of serotonergic (5-HT) activity in the brain.

The relationship between altered serotonergic activity and depression is discussed further below. However, there is also evidence linking carbohydrate craving to 5-HT activity in the brain (Spring *et al.* 1987). Tryptophan, the precursor of 5-HT, is only available from dietary protein. It competes with other amino-acids for transport into the brain. Paradoxically a protein meal decreases, whereas a carbohydrate meal increases, brain tryptophan. This is probably because the carbohydrate meal triggers greater insulin release, as a result of which most of the other amino-acids in the blood, apart from tryptophan, are taken up by muscle, leaving the transport system, used to transfer amino acids across the blood–brain barrier, free to transport tryptophan (Fernstrom & Wurtman, 1971). Thus, carbohydrate-rich meals, by increasing the availability of tryptophan in the brain, enhance the synthesis and release of 5-HT, as indicated by increased levels of the 5-HT metabolite, 5-hydroxyindoleacetic acid (5-HIAA), in the CSF (Fernstrom & Wurtman, 1972).

It has been postulated that the increased carbohydrate intake of women with premenstrual depression is a form of self-medication to counteract the adverse effect of 5-HT depletion on mood. Dalton & Holton (1992) advocate 3-hourly carbohydrate intake as a method of self-management of premenstrual symptoms, and claim that a proportion of women benefit substantially. Wurtman *et al.* (1989) found that PMS sufferers who consumed a high carbohydrate/low protein meal, in experimental circumstances, experienced substantial improvements in depressed mood. A similar effect was reported in subjects with Seasonal Affective Disorder, a form of depression typically associated with increased appetite (Rosenthal *et al.* 1986). (Major depressive illness is typically associated with loss of appetite.) However, Hill *et al.* (1991) found that in non-PMS sufferers, when sweet-food craving occurred in the presence of depressed mood, responding to the craving by eating carbohydrates led to a continuation of the depressed mood, whereas resisting the craving was followed by some mood improvement.

Obviously, the reaction to food craving, whatever its links to brain biochemistry, is going to be influenced by psychological mechanisms. In particular, premenstrual food craving is often experienced, by women who feel depressed premenstrually, as a further threat to their sense of self-control and self-esteem. Bowen & Grunberg (1990) studied the relevance of 'eating restraint', a psychological characteristic, and found that 'high restraint' women with premenstrual craving suffered more premenstrual symptoms than those with low restraint.

In a recent study of insulin-dependent diabetic women who regarded themselves as PMS sufferers (Cawood *et al.* 1993), those who reported premenstrual food craving were more likely to experience reduction in diabetic control during the premenstrual and menstrual phases, with increased glucose in the blood or urine, presumably a consequence of increased carbohydrate intake. According to the Fernstrom & Wurtman hypothesis (1971), the benefit of the carbohydrate intake depends on the consequences of the induced release of insulin. In the insulin-dependent diabetic woman, no such insulin release should occur and hence the effect on mood should be different. The diabetic woman with premenstrual food craving may provide a useful opportunity for testing this hypothesis.

Premenstrual food craving does appear to be a cycle-related phenomenon which is both common and of potential theoretical importance. However, it remains to be demonstrated that its occurrence is a consequence of depleted brain 5-HT activity, and further studies of the effects of carbohydrate intake on mood will need to take into account the psychological complexities of 'giving in to craving'. If its link to 5-HT is established, cycle-related food craving will be a valuable marker to explore the impact of the ovarian cycle on women's well-being and mood. It is also of interest that D-fenfluramine, an appetite suppressant which increases 5-HT release and inhibits its re-uptake in the CNS, has been shown both to reduce carbohydrate intake and improve mood in women with premenstrual depression (Brzezinski *et al.* 1990). This finding, which requires replication, also offers therapeutic possibilities.

### G. Physical changes

The two most common cycle-related physical changes reported by PMS sufferers are 'bloating' and breast swelling and tenderness. In two large-scale epidemiological studies, breast swelling was reported by 50 to 60% of women, and abdominal bloating by 60 to 70%.

Up to 60% of women experience some breast pain, usually during the luteal phase (Mansel, 1988), and in a survey of women attending a breast-screening unit, 69% of premenopausal and perimenopausal women reported cyclical breast pain, becoming more common with age (Leinster *et al.* 1987). The mechanisms underlying this common cyclical breast change have received little attention and are not well understood. Milligan *et al.* (1975) reported that during normal ovarian cycles the volume increase in the breast was confined to the luteal phase, whereas in o.c. cycles it occurs throughout the 21 days of o.c. administration. Ayers & Gidwani (1983) compared 25 women with cyclical breast pain and 15 asymptomatic controls. The two groups did not differ in the prevalence of fibrocystic disease (FCD), as shown by ultrasound, but there were endocrine differences between the groups. The breast pain group showed similar levels of oestradiol but significantly lower progesterone levels than the controls in the mid-luteal phase. They also showed greater prolactin response to TRH. These hormonal differences were not related to the presence or absence of FCD. The progesterone differences are reminiscent of some early findings of deficient luteal phase levels of progesterone in women with PMS. Clearly this interesting study should be replicated, with particular emphasis on women experiencing perimenstrual mood change, and comparing those with and without premenstrual breast pain.

Physiological mechanisms underlying the various forms of bloating, such as abdominal bloating and the less common finger swelling, have also received little research attention. Whereas these symptoms are widely attributed to fluid retention, leading to the use of diuretics for treatment, there is little evidence of fluid retention or weight gain in the large majority of women with this complaint (Bancroft & Bäckström, 1985). A discrepancy between perceived and actual body size is apparent (Faratian *et al.* 1984) and requires explanation. There is some evidence of an alteration in capillary permeability through the cycle (Jones *et al.* 1966; Wong *et al.* 1972). Interstitial fluid volume increases if transcapillary filtration rate is greater than the lymph flow. This filtration rate is regulated by both the colloid osmotic pressure and hydrostatic pressure in the plasma and interstitial fluid. Oian *et al.* (1987) found a fall in the colloid osmotic pressure of both the plasma and the interstitial fluid from the follicular to luteal phase. Although the women in this study were not suffering from PMS, this change in fluid dynamics could underly the cyclical experience of bloatedness. There may be comparable effects within the mesenteric vascular bed contributing to abdominal bloating. However, many women report alteration of bowel habit during the luteal phase, and some degree of gaseous distension or altered sensitivity of the bowel wall may be contributing.

## H. Neurotransmitter activity in the CNS

The direct effects of ovarian steroids on cellular activity within the CNS has been demonstrated in rodents, with oestradiol having an excitatory and progesterone an inhibitory effect. Such effects, which are probably mediated by membrane action of the steroids rather than by genomic effects, are consistent with the variation in frequency of certain kinds of epileptic seizures through the human menstrual cycle. But the relevance of such cellular mechanisms to cycle-related changes in well-being and mood remains unknown (Bancroft & Bäckström, 1985).

Of the various central neurotransmitters that may be implicated in the control of mood and mood disorders, 5-HT and noradrenaline (NA) are receiving the most attention at the present time. The question of whether such neurotransmitters normally vary in activity through the ovarian cycle is therefore relevant to the mild variation in well-being that many women experience.

The effects of ovarian steroids on neurotransmitter function within the CNS has been studied in some detail in the rodent. However, it is not possible, even in the rodent, to describe a general pattern of change in neurotransmitter function through the reproductive cycle. Levels of neurotransmitters and related enzymes, such as monoamine oxidase (MAO), change differentially depending on the brain area examined, reflecting the various functions that neurotransmitters serve (Luine & McEwen, 1985). Thus, Biegon *et al.* (1980) assayed the 5-HT receptor levels in different brain regions of the rat at different stages of the oestrous cycle. In the cortex and caudate no differences across the cycle were found. In the basal forebrain (including hypothalamus, septum and pre-optic area), receptor levels were 40% lower during pro-oestrous and oestrous (when oestrogen levels are high) than during di-oestrous (when oestrogen is low). As 5-HT has a predominantly inhibitory effect on rodent sexual behaviour, they interpreted this effect as an oestrogenic facilitation of oestrous sexual behaviour. In relation to perimenstrual mood change in women, it is postulated that there is a decline in 5-HT activity in the late luteal and early follicular phase when oestradiol levels are low. This illustrates the problems in extrapolating from rodent to human in this context.

In any case, the opportunities for studying steroid-neurotransmitter interaction in the human are much more limited, largely confined to (a) measuring levels of neurotransmitter and related enzymes, or of platelet receptor levels and binding dynamics in the plasma, at different stages of the cycle, and (b) neuroendocrine challenge tests which are mediated by neurotransmitters and carried out at different stages of the cycle. Measuring circulating levels of neurotransmitters, apart from being methodologically difficult, tells us nothing about variations in neurotransmitter activity in specific areas of the brain. Neuroendocrine challenge tests do have the advantage of testing a specific response system in the CNS. Both types of evidence, limited in amount, will be considered.

### I. Circulating levels of neurotransmitter

Monoamine oxidase (MAO), the principal enzyme in the degradation of catecholamines, has been measured in relation to the menstrual cycle, with inconsistent results. Two studies have shown an increase of platelet MAO activity around ovulation, declining in the luteal phase (Belmaker *et al.* 1974; Baron *et al.* 1980), another study reporting the opposite pattern (Poirier *et al.* 1985).

Platelets have also been widely used to assess levels of 5-HT receptors, usually with tritiated imipramine as the ligand. Poirier *et al.* (1986) found no variation in such binding at weekly intervals in 10 normal women. In a further study (Peters *et al.* 1979), neither 5-HT or NA receptors were found to vary through the normal cycle, whereas there were significant differences between day 21 and day 28, in both types of receptor, in women taking oral contraceptives.

Ashby *et al.* (1988) compared 10 PMS sufferers and 10 controls. In neither group were there any significant differences between premenstrual and postmenstrual parameters of 5-HT platelet affinity and uptake (Km and Vmax). However, the Vmax was significantly lower in the PMS group than the controls during the premenstrual phase. Rapkin *et al.* (1987) measured whole-blood 5-HT levels in 14 PMS sufferers and 13 age-matched controls. The interesting finding in this study was that 5-HT levels in the PMS group remained unaltered through the cycle, whereas in the controls they rose during the luteal phase to their highest level premenstrually. The two groups were not significantly different during the follicular phase, but the controls did show higher 5-HT levels during the luteal phase. Tam *et al.* (1985) studied platelet 5-HT uptake in 6 women without premenstrual mood change and found that both Km and Vmax were significantly higher on day 24 of the cycle than on days 1 to 10. Taylor *et al.* (1984) found lower levels of plasma 5-HT premenstrually than postmenstrually in 16 women with PMS; 5-HT binding parameters also correlated with ratings of some premenstrual symptoms. No controls were involved in this study.

It is not possible from these results to conclude that there is any predictable change in 5-HT activity through the cycle in normal women. The evidence is more suggestive of a change in PMS sufferers, and the interesting possibility from one study (Rapkin *et al.* 1987), that there is a compensatory increase in circulating 5-HT during the luteal phase which perhaps protects the 'non-PMS' woman from premenstrual mood change, and which is relatively lacking in women prone to such mood change, might warrant further study.

### J. Neuroendocrine challenge tests

Clonidine, an alpha-2 adrenoceptor agonist, elicits a GH response which is typically blunted in depressive illness (Cowen & Anderson, 1991). This response was found to be blunted during menstruation in normal women (Matussek *et al.* 1984).

Intravenous L-tryptophan, the precursor of 5-HT, produces a prolactin (PRL) response which is typically blunted in depressive illness (Cowen & Anderson, 1991). This response was found to be significantly less premenstrually (days −1 to −4) than postmenstrually (days +8 to +14) in both controls and women with perimenstrual depression (Bancroft *et al.* 1991). Best *et al.* (1992) assessing the effect of oestradiol on the L-tryptophan challenge, found the prolactin response to be significantly increased after an oestradiol implant in oophorectomized women.

D-fenfluramine is a specific 5-HT releasing and re-uptake blocking agent which stimulates PRL release in normal subjects, a response which tends to be blunted in depressed subjects. D-fenfluramine challenge (30 mg) was given at three stages of the cycle: early follicular (days 1 to 3), mid-cycle (days 12 to 14) and late luteal (days 24 to 26), in 9 normal women (O'Keane *et al.* 1991). The PRL response differed considerably for these three phases, being maximal mid-cycle and minimal in the early follicular phase.

This pattern was reflected in the oestradiol levels. However, Bancroft *et al.* (1993*b*) assessed the response to D-fenfluramine (15 mg or 30 mg according to body weight) at two stages of the cycle – premenstrually (days −2 to −5) and postmenstrually (days 9 to 13, median day 10) in 11 women with no premenstrual mood change. Prolactin responses were clearly evident on both occasions and did not differ significantly. It is possible that the failure to find the postmenstrual increase reported in the previous study was because of a slightly earlier timing of the postmenstrual test, more likely to miss the relatively short-lived pre-ovulatory rise in oestradiol.

The receptor sub-type mediation of these effects of different 5-HT agonists is likely to be complex. Cowen (1992) has summarized the evidence concluding, on the basis of specific receptor antagonist studies, that the prolactin and GH responses to L-tryptophan are mediated by post-synaptic $5\text{-HT}_{1A}$ receptors. The cortisol response to L-tryptophan has been less studied (and appears to be less predictable). The cortisol response to 5-hydroxytryptophan is apparently more predictable and the limited evidence suggests that this response is mediated by post-synaptic $5\text{-HT}_2$ receptors. With D-fenfluramine, a GH response is not expected and the prolactin response appears to be mediated via $5\text{-HT}_{2/1c}$ receptors. While this picture remains unclear and difficult to explain, variations in neuro-endocrine response to difference 5-HT agonists should not be surprising.

Dinan *et al.* (1990) reported the prolactin response to buspirone in 6 female volunteers during the follicular, mid-cycle and luteal phases (the precise timing of these phases was not given). The prolactin response was highest in the luteal phase. However, while buspirone is predominantly a $5\text{-HT}_{1A}$ agonist, it also has dopaminergic effects which are likely to confound the prolactin response (Anderson, 1989).

Therefore, we have limited evidence consistent with there being an alteration in 5-HT activity perimenstrually, a pattern which may be relevant to the 'timing factor'. However, a crucial question remains unanswered. If, as seems likely, the varying responses through the cycle, particularly to 5-HT agonists, reflect varying levels of oestradiol we have two possible explanations to consider. One is that oestradiol influences neurotransmitter activity in the CNS which is reflected in the pituitary response; this effect would be of direct relevance to our subject. An alternative explanation is that oestrogen enhances the PRL response to a variety of stimuli (e.g. Buckman *et al.* 1976), by direct effects on the lactotroph. If so, variations in prolactin response through the cycle could simply be a function of this oestrogenic effect on the pituitary and hence of less interest to our subject. Assessing the impact of the cycle on the prolactin response to more direct pituitary challenges might help to resolve this issue. However, once again the evidence is inconsistent. Cycle-related changes in PRL response to TRH were observed in one study (Boyd & Sanchez-Franco, 1976) but not in others (McNeilly & Hagen, 1974; Roy-Byrne *et al.* 1987; Casper *et al.* 1989). Also, Tan *et al.* (1986) found that, whereas the PRL response to gonadotrophin releasing hormone (GnRH) was greater in the luteal than the early follicular phases of normally cycling women, the response in postmenopausal women, whose oestrogen levels were low, was greater than the early follicular phase responses of the pre-menopausal women.

Some doubt about the determinants of the PRL response to neuroendocrine challenge therefore remain and need to be resolved before it can be used as an index of varying neuro-transmitter activity in the CNS.

## VI. THE MENSTRUATION FACTOR

### A. The control of menstruation

As with the ovarian cycle, the physiology of menstrual bleeding is incompletely understood, particularly the mechanisms which determine the onset of bleeding (Brenner & Maslar, 1988). However, a crucial factor, for the normal menstrual cycle, is the imposition of the effects of luteal phase progesterone on the continuing stimulatory effects of oestradiol. During the luteal or secretory phase of the cycle, the glandular structures in the endometrium become more active. From 7 to 8 days before the onset of bleeding, the endometrial stroma becomes oedematous, and the stromal cells surrounding the spiral arteries hypertrophy and show increased mitotic activity. (The spiral arterioles are a characteristic feature of the endometrium in those few species, such as the human, where endometrial shedding and menstruation occurs.) This is accompanied by first lymphocyte and later neutrophil infiltration suggestive of a local inflammatory reaction. Shortly before bleeding starts there is a reabsorption of fluid, with substantial shrinkage of the tissue, and increasing evidence of cell death. This is believed to be a form of apoptosis (programmed cell death) triggered by the falling levels of progesterone.

The stromal shrinkage leads to increased coiling of the spiral arteries, and is accompanied by vascular stasis. There is then, over a period varying from 4 to 24 h, a recurrent cycle of vasodilatation followed by intense vasoconstriction which eventually results in the onset of bleeding.

Prostaglandins (PGs) are believed to contribute to this process (Abel, 1985). $PGF2\alpha$ probably induces the vasoconstriction and spasm. This PG is produced in increasing amounts in the endometrium towards the end of the luteal phase as progesterone levels fall. PGE2 on the other hand is a modest vasodilator. $PGF2\alpha$ is the principal PG to be secreted by the endometrium, but the ratio of $PGF2\alpha$ and PGE2 does vary in ways which may have clinical significance. $PGF2\alpha$ tends to be increased in the endometrium and menstrual fluid in women with primary dysmenorrhoea, and in general PGs have been shown to be hyperalgesic, whereas increased PGE2 is found in women with heavy blood loss. However, the precise role of these PGs in the control of menstruation is not yet established. Prostaglandin synthetase inhibitors (e.g. mefenamic acid), for example, may reduce heavy blood loss but have little effect on more moderate flow. There is no doubt that there is a variable degree of build up of not only the various PGs but other relatively toxic substances such as cytokines and activated oxygen species, in the endometrium during the luteal phase, some of which may well escape into the general circulation to have more distant effects.

There are many other crucial questions which wait to be answered. For example, it is not understood what mechanisms are involved in the initiation of bleeding in anovular cycles when there is no substantial rise and fall of progesterone.

When we consider the woman's experience of menstruation, there are two contrasting and possibly conflicting aspects to consider. The first concerns the relief of symptoms which often occurs with the onset of menstrual bleeding – we can call this the 'menstrual relief' effect. The second, mentioned earlier, concerns the possible ways in which disturbed menstruation may aggravate the mood changes and other symptoms which occur perimenstrually.

## B. Menstrual relief

The classical description of PMS involves the relief of symptoms with the onset of menstrual bleeding. Some women give a vivid description of this effect; e.g. 'I know when my period has started even before I go to the toilet because I feel a weight lifting off my shoulders'. Often the temporal relationship is not quite as dramatic as this, but there is considerable relief during the first day of menstrual bleeding. The proportion of women suffering from premenstrual changes who experience this clearcut change with the onset of bleeding is not known. It is reported by a small proportion of women who attend our PMS clinic. Rather more women describe how this used to be the case, but with time their symptoms have taken longer and longer to remit after the start of bleeding. In some cases, symptoms are present for most of the cycle but there is a short-lived remission with the onset of bleeding with the early return of symptoms either before the end of the menstrual phase or soon after. This is sometimes the case in women with chronic depression.

Another description which is not unusual is from the woman whose cycles are irregular, and who has prolonged cycles some of the time. She may describe how the symptoms start at the usual time but menstruation is delayed and the severity of symptoms builds up until bleeding finally begins. In such circumstances the woman longs for the start of her period. Our assessment of women who are established on oral contraceptives when they complain of PMS has led us to recognize at least two contrasting patterns. In some women, symptoms only occur during the pill-free interval and can sometimes be avoided or delayed by extending the length of the pill cycle. They can be regarded as a form of 'withdrawal' symptoms. In others, the symptoms start well before the end of the pill phase to be relieved when bleeding starts – examples of 'menstrual relief'. In such women we have sometimes avoided the usual severity of symptoms by instituting a short pill cycle (e.g. 17 days of pill and 5 days pill-free interval) which cuts short the development of symptoms (McNeill, 1992). With observations of this kind it is difficult to avoid the conclusion that in some way mechanisms involved in the initiation of menstrual bleeding produce a relief of symptoms. Obviously it is difficult to separate the onset of bleeding itself from the falling steroid levels which are likely to precede it. But the remarkable coincidence of bleeding onset and symptom relief in some cases at least raises the possibility that there is a mechanism other than falling steroid levels which contributes to the relief. Is it possible that a build-up of 'toxic' metabolites such as cytokines and activated oxygen species, or hyperalgesic prostaglandins such as PGE2, occurs in the endometrium, resulting in release of these substances into the circulation *until* menstrual flow starts? (I am grateful to Dr Rodney Kelly for this interesting suggestion.) If so, the 'old wives tale' that menstrual bleeding 'cleans' the blood may not be as wide of the mark as is normally assumed.

## C. Menstrual aggravation

The other aspect is probably much more common and clinically important – the extent to which menstruation may aggravate perimenstrual symptoms. This can be considered at two levels – the direct effects of pain, and the more indirect effects of changes associated with the build-up and shedding of the endometrium on other parts of the body, including the central nervous system. We will consider this aspect under three headings: (i) the effects of pain; (ii) the possible relevance of cyclical changes in prostaglandin production; and (iii) the impact of hysterectomy on 'perimenstrual' symptoms.

### (i) Dysmenorrhoea

Although a number of studies have identified a relationship between dysmenorrhoea and premenstrual symptoms, it is striking how little attention has been given to the relevance of pain in the PMS literature. Coppen & Kessell (1963) found not only that dysmenorrhoea was correlated with premenstrual syndrome, but also when women reported both complaints, the pain was more likely to start during the premenstrual phase. Wood *et al.* (1979) also found a strong association between dysmenorrhoea and premenstrual tension in a large group of women attending a health testing centre. In a study of women attending a premenstrual syndrome clinic, Steege *et al.* (1985) found the severity of premenstrual symptoms was correlated with the severity of dysmenorrhoea. A similar relationship was reported by women attending a community health centre (Graham & Sherwin, 1987). Dalton (1984) has presented a confusing picture. On the one hand, she regards painless menstruation as a characteristic of premenstrual syndrome (p. 33); on the other hand, she equates 'congestive dysmenorrhoea', in which pain starts premenstrually, with premenstrual syndrome: 'In this group pain is a prominent symptom of their premenstrual syndrome and increases in intensity until the onset of the full menstrual flow' (p. 185).

In our clinic study discussed earlier, (Bancroft *et al.* 1993*b*) not only was mood change, both premenstrual and menstrual, evident in the large majority of women presenting with dysmenorrhoea, most of these women reported their period-type pain starting in the premenstrual phase. This association can be explained at a relatively simple psychological level. In women who recurrently experience disabling dysmenorrhoea, the anticipation of pain may well induce negative mood as menstruation approaches. Similarly, in the presence of such pain, lowered mood would not be surprising. However, it may be premature to accept such an explanation as sufficient. Are other mechanisms involved?

Menstrual pain is typically associated with uterine contractions. While these contractions are maximal in intensity during menstrual flow, they occur during the luteal phase of the cycle, depending on the hormonal milieu, gradually building up to the pattern associated with menstrual bleeding (Hein, 1975). Painful uterine contractions have been shown to be associated with high levels of endometrial prostaglandin production. The associated pain is believed to be, in part, a result of myometrial ischaemia (Ulmsten, 1985). Although primary dysmenorrhoea is typically regarded as being confined to the menstrual phase, starting no more than a few hours before the onset of menstrual flow, little research has been done on the characteristics of period-type pain which while unassociated with obvious pelvic pathology, such as endometriosis, nevertheless starts several days before the onset of bleeding. It is a reasonable assumption that in such cases, for whatever reasons, high levels of endometrial prostaglandins are being produced.

### (*ii*) *The role of prostaglandins*

Prostaglandins are 'local hormones' synthesized in virtually all tissues, more so in certain types of cell such as the macrophage. Their universal presence can perhaps be most economically explained in terms of local mediation of immune and inflammatory mechanisms; hence their important role in the causation of pain. Their role in the uterus may be an example of specialized functional development. Similarly in the CNS specialized functions may have evolved, such as the control of hypothalamic–pituitary hormone release. In general they are very difficult substances to study in vivo because their local production is easily affected by experimental manipulation of tissue. Also they are rapidly metabolized, not only by the lungs, but also by the uterus, so that measurement of circulating levels is of little value. However, it is plausible that prostaglandins could be contributing to a variety of symptoms associated with premenstrual syndrome as a result of their local action e.g. pain induction or lowered threshold to pain, vasodilatation (Craig, 1980; Bancroft & Bäckström, 1985).

One approach to evaluating their role is to assess the effect of prostaglandin synthetase inhibiting drugs, such as aspirin or mefenamic acid, in relieving the symptoms of PMS. We have limited and inconclusive evidence of this kind. Wood & Jakubowicz (1980) studied the effects of mefenamic acid (500 mg *t.i.d.*) in 37 women in a placebo-controlled cross-over design. It was noteworthy in this study that most women had menstrual symptoms (e.g. pain) as well as premenstrual. Symptoms in both phases, including irritability and depression, were improved; breast tenderness was notable in not responding. Here there was evidence that if menstrual symptoms such as dysmenorrhoea are relieved by prostaglandin synthetase inhibitors, other perimenstrual symptoms are also improved. Unfortunately little consideration was given to the possibility that the primary effect of treatment was on the pain. A further study was carried out which was less informative than the first; no assessment of menstrual symptoms such as pain was reported, and the method of assessing improvement was not described (Jakubowicz *et al.* 1984). The best study from the methodological point of view was by Mira *et al.* (1986). Only 15 women were involved in a placebo-controlled cross over design, starting with mefenamic acid (250 mg *t.i.d.*) from day 16, increasing to 500 mg *t.i.d.* from day 19. Significant improvement was reported in a number of premenstrual symptoms, in particular fatigue, headaches and general aches and pains, and to a lesser extent, negative mood change. Once again little attention was paid to the presence and contribution of menstrual symptoms such as pain. All the reader is told is that women were only included in the study if they had 'no evidence of gynaecologic disease, for example recurrent herpes genitalis, menorrhagia or severe dysmenorrhoea'. No details were given of how menorrhagia or severe dysmenorrhoea were defined. Furthermore, the report was flawed by the absence of any actual symptom ratings – results were presented simply in terms of significance levels, which makes the clinical relevance of the observed effects impossible to evaluate.

Nevertheless, these studies lend some support to the notion of prostaglandins *at least contributing* to the symptom complex of PMS. If they are playing such a role we are left with a fundamental conundrum: are these effects the result of prostaglandins produced by the uterus and released into the circulation or are they derived locally, in various parts of the body including the CNS, stimulated by the same pattern of ovarian steroids that are responsible for the build up of endometrial prostaglandins? One obvious approach to answering the conundrum is to assess the effects of hysterectomy in women whose ovaries are conserved; they at least will have their uterine source of prostaglandins removed.

### (*iii*) *The effects of hysterectomy*

Bäckström *et al.* (1981) reported a careful study of 7 women with established PMS who were about to undergo hysterectomy. Cyclical symptoms returned reaching their maximum during the luteal phase of the subsequent ovarian cycles. This was important evidence of the relationship between cyclical symptoms and hormonal changes uncomplicated by the effects of menstruation. There was also a 'small but significant improvement' in these symptoms following hysterectomy. In terms of global symptom ratings, this reduction was 40 % in the late luteal phase ($P < 0.025$) and 33 % ($P < 0.025$) during the early follicular (menstrual) phase.

Osborn & Gath (1990) assessed 56 women before and after hysterectomy. No attempt was made to select women who were experiencing significant premenstrual symptoms. While this study involved much effort, it is difficult to interpret. A comparison is made of '5 premenstrual days' and the 'remaining intermenstrual days'. Presumably menstrual days were excluded, though this was not made clear, and given that all these women were experiencing menstrual problems, menstrual days could have taken up much of the cycle for many of them. Symptom severity during the menstrual days was ignored. Post-hysterectomy, the 'five premenstrual days' were based on an assessment of the ovarian cycle and an estimation of when menstrual bleeding would have occurred if an intact uterus had been present. The 'intermenstrual days', post-operatively, were presumably the rest of the cycle. The possibility that 'five bad days' might have been occurring elsewhere in the ovarian cycle was not considered. The authors' principal conclusion, that because of a reduction in 'premenstrual symptoms' post-operatively, the pre-operative premenstrual symptoms must have been psychologically rather than biologically determined, is quite unjustified. However, these results do lend some support to the idea that the physical and emotional well-being of women 'premenstrually' is adversely affected by severe menstrual problems, and hence improves after hysterectomy. While the hysterectomy model is an interesting one, the interpretation of symptom levels pre- and post-operation must take into account the morbidity that led to the hysterectomy in the first place.

Metcalf *et al.* (1991) used a different approach. They recruited 44 women who had undergone hysterectomy and who believed that they still experienced cyclical symptoms, comparable to the premenstrual changes they had experienced pre-operatively. They carefully assessed the timing of cyclical symptoms in relation to the ovarian cycle in these women, the majority of whom did show cyclical patterns, and compared these patterns with those of women with intact uteri. They used their normative hormonal data to establish when the hysterectomized women would have started to bleed if they had had a uterus (in a manner comparable to that of Osborne & Gath, 1990). They found that the peak of symptoms, both emotional and physical, occurred significantly earlier (by 2·5 days on average) in the hormonal cycles of the hysterectomized women. This interesting finding casts further doubt on Osborn & Gath's conclusions (i.e. they probably looked at the wrong five days!). It also led Metcalf and her colleagues to suggest that menstruation in some way alters the timing and/or severity of premenstrual symptoms. There is more than one explanation for such an effect; the timing of the peak could be simply delayed in intact women; alternatively, the contribution of the ovarian cycle (what we have earlier called the 'timing factor') could be relatively early but the shape of the 'peak' altered by the addition of the aggravating influences of menstruation on the premenstrual phase, giving the impression of a later peak.

Metcalf *et al.* (1992) subsequently examined a group of 12 PMS sufferers before and after hysterectomy. Ten of the 12 women showed a reduction in their emotional symptom severity post-operatively. In addition to this, there was also a change in the timing of peaks of symptoms. Whereas most women continued to show significant peaks of symptoms, pre-operatively most of these had clustered around the '92%' point of the cycle (taking 100% as the end of the cycle). Post-operatively, these peaks were much more widely scattered. These authors considered several possible explanations for such changes. They found no evidence of an alteration of ovarian function post-operatively. A 'tonic' effect of the operation, producing a general improvement in well-being, could have contributed to the improvement. They compared the six women whose general health was markedly improved following the surgery with the remainder whose general health showed little improvement. There were no systematic differences in the changes in cycle-related symptoms in these two sub-groups, leading them to conclude that the 'tonic' effect was not important. Altered expectations and the 'placebo' effect of the surgery were also considered. It so happened that three of the women had been involved in a study evaluating the effects of placebo before undergoing surgery. Their symptom reduction post-operatively was somewhat greater than that in response to placebo treatment. Obviously, it is difficult to control for such effects and they may well contribute to the overall improvement. However, an earlier study by this group (Metcalf & Hudson, 1985) had shown a general tendency for symptom peaks to be delayed in the ovarian cycle when responding to placebo, whereas following surgery they were by comparison scattered, or in the larger study (Metcalf *et al.* 1991), earlier in the hormonal cycle.

The evidence so far therefore points to an influence of the uterus and the processes of menstruation on the experience of premenstrual as well as menstrual phase symptoms. This suggests that if prostaglandins are important, they are at least in part coming from the uterus. Placebo-controlled studies of prostaglandin-synthetase inhibitors in women experiencing cyclical symptoms *after hysterectomy*, would be an effective way of assessing the importance of extra-uterine prostaglandins. Further research of this kind is required to throw more light on the 'menstruation factor'. The post-hysterectomy model also offers a number of opportunities, for example the assessment of the 'timing factor' uncomplicated by the effects of menstruation.

## VII. THE VULNERABILITY FACTOR

If changes occur within the CNS which are related to the ovarian cycle, why are some women more susceptible to these changes than others? This is the issue of 'vulnerability', which may reflect the current circumstances that a woman faces, such as adverse life events and other sources of stress, as well as characteristics of the woman herself, which are not in themselves functions of the menstrual cycle but which influence or determine how she will react to and cope with her menstrual cycle-related changes.

Evidence that menstrual symptoms were worse during stressful life experiences was reported by Siegel *et al.* (1979), though this association was less marked in women using o.c.s. Although this association conformed with clinical experience, there is as yet no systematic attempt to relate premenstrual symptoms in clinic attenders to the levels and types of current adversity they are experiencing.

The characteristics of the woman which contribute to such vulnerability can be conceptualized, as follows, in a variety of ways.

(*i*) *Cognitive style*   Are there ways of thinking which render some women more susceptible to cyclical mood changes? Recent interest in the use of cognitive therapy in the treatment of PMS has highlighted this aspect (e.g. Morse & Dennerstein, 1988).

(*ii*) *Attitudes to menstruation* These and other negative expectations which a woman learns from her culture, are often cited as important determinants of how she experiences menstruation. As yet there is little evidence that such factors contribute much to the more distressing forms of perimenstrual mood changes.

(*iii*) *Personality*   This is a global term, which covers the variety of ways in which an individual *typically* reacts to circumstances, including her usual repertoire of coping strategies. 'Neuroticism' is a dimension of personality which has been linked to PMS in a number of studies (Coppen & Kessel, 1963; Mira *et al.* 1985; Bancroft *et al.* 1993*a*). As discussed earlier, it may be especially relevant to patterns of help-seeking behaviour, as well as a predisposition for emotional problems. As such it is certainly relevant to our concept of vulnerability.

(*iv*) *Autonomic reactivity* An individual's typical pattern of psychophysiological response to stressful situations which in itself may lead to further anxiety or stress (e.g. the feedback effects of increased heart rate).

(*v*) *Propensity for depressive illness*   A complex product of genetic, early constitutional and situational factors (e.g. current levels of adversity).

(*vi*) *Capacity for biological adaptation* The ability to adjust to neurobiological change to maintain stability. If changes in neurotransmitters occur as a result of the ovarian cycle, vulnerability may reflect an inability to compensate for or correct such changes.

While in many respects conceptually distinct, these headings can be regarded as different views or 'windows' into the complexity of the human condition – reflecting the 'state' model of Wolff mentioned earlier. To consider all of these 'windows' of vulnerability in any depth is well beyond the scope of this review, and would need to embrace a vast literature. However, the neurobiological dimension is of particular relevance. This confronts us with the difference between a 'trait', reflecting the individual's typical way of responding and a 'state', i.e. the current status of the individual's response system. As yet, our knowledge of 'trait' markers of a neurobiological nature is very limited. We are in a better position with respect to 'state' markers, particularly in relation to the 'state' of depressed mood, and we will consider the neurobiological aspects of the state of depression more closely below. The reason why 'state' biological markers are also important to this discussion, is because they may enable us to comprehend an interaction between a 'state' in this sense and some transitory change of function imposed by the ovarian cycle. The changes normally associated with the ovarian cycle may be of little consequence to a woman when she is in her normal 'state', but may interact with an abnormal 'state' to result in significant mood change perimenstrually.

## A. The link between PMS and depressive illness

The possibility that women who suffer from PMS are more at risk for major depressive disorder has been a contentious issue for some years. This link is largely based on studies in which current PMS status, usually determined crudely by means of retrospective ratings, has been associated with a past history of depressive illness, also based on retrospective assessment, often covering a long time period (Kashiwagi *et al.* 1976; Endicott *et al.* 1985; Halbreich & Endicott, 1985*b*; Mackenzie *et al.* 1986; Stout *et al.* 1986; Warner *et al.* 1991). The link, if real, is of potentially great importance; it would enable the recognition of those at risk for future major depressive disorder. Furthermore, if the recurrence of perimenstrual changes leads to more chronic depression, this might help to explain the substantial sex difference in the prevalence of depressive illness. It also raises the possibility that recurrent short-term perimenstrual mood changes provide us, in some sense, with a model of major depression, allowing neurobiological as well as psychological studies which are difficult if not impossible in states of chronic depressive illness.

However, this link remains tenuous. DeJong *et al.* (1985), in one of the few studies in which

links between current PMS and past depressive illness were studied by means of prospective assessment of PMS status, threw doubt on the link. Among women who regarded themselves as PMS sufferers, the association with past history was more marked in those who did not meet the prospective criteria for PMS, than in those who did. Our recent studies in Edinburgh have thrown some light on this puzzle. A past history of depression, treated with antidepressants, was found to be associated to some extent with the likelihood of experiencing premenstrual onset of depressive mood, but more markedly with the duration of such depressive mood once initiated. Women with such depressive histories were more likely to report depressive mood that persisted through the menstrual phase and sometimes for a few days into the postmenstrual phase (Warner *et al.* 1991). This association was also found in a subsequent study, using the same methods of assessment (Bancroft *et al.* 1993*c*). This could account for some of the earlier confusion, because this tendency for more prolonged perimenstrual mood change, in women with a history of depressive illness, reduces the likelihood of their meeting the arbitrary criteria for PMS – further powerful support for the critique of such criteria presented earlier in this review.

These findings therefore suggest that a past history of depression is especially relevant to our concept of vulnerability; it may increase the likelihood of experiencing premenstrual mood change in the first place, but it is particularly likely to influence the duration and possibly the severity of that mood change if and when it occurs. Is it possible that this form of vulnerability to menstrual cycle changes may depend on neurobiological factors which characterize the woman with a past history of depressive illness?

In general, we have little information about neurobiological characteristics which distinguish people who are prone to depression *when they are not depressed*. In other words, the evidence that we do have is probably of the 'state' rather than 'trait' variety, obtained from people who are either in the midst of a depressive illness or in the process of recovering from it or entering into it. It is nevertheless of interest to ask whether such biological markers of depressive illness are present in women who suffer from perimenstrual depression, either during the premenstrual phase of their cycle or at any stage of the cycle, reflecting their current 'state' of vulnerability.

The neurobiological markers of depressive illness which have received the most attention can be considered under four headings: (i) alteration of sleep pattern; (ii) levels of receptors for neurotransmitters, such as 5-HT or noradrenaline, which may be implicated in depressive states; (iii) response to neuroendocrine challenge tests; and (iv) the function of the hypothalamo–pituitary–adrenal axis.

### (i) Sleep and sleep-related hormonal activity

Alterations of sleep pattern, such as reduced latency of REM-phase sleep, are now well established as characteristics of depressive illness, though their functional significance is not yet understood. Their possible link to alterations of biological rhythms led to the 'phase advance' hypothesis of depression (Wehr *et al.* 1979).

We have very little evidence of sleep pattern in women with perimenstrual mood changes. Parry *et al.* (1989) studied sleep and body temperature at intervals throughout the cycle in 8 women with premenstrual depression and 8 controls. Only two differences were observed; a greater amount of Stage 2 and less REM sleep in the women with premenstrual mood change. These differences were not confined to the premenstrual phase and were not characteristic of major depressive illness. Their significance is not understood and, with such small numbers, further evidence of this kind is required.

In a further study, (Parry *et al.* 1990) nocturnal secretion of melatonin was measured, again in 8 patients with PMS and 8 controls. The patients had an earlier offset of melatonin secretion, contributing to a shorter duration of secretion. This can be regarded as an example of 'phase advance' of the sleep–wake cycle. Once again this abnormality was present throughout the cycle and was not confined to the premenstrual or late luteal phase. According to these authors, such changes may reflect some disruption of the melatonin-mediated entrainment of the circadian rhythm by the environment (e.g. light–dark cycle) of possible relevance to the causation of both depressive illness and PMS.

Total sleep deprivation improves mood in depressive illness, at least until the next period of sleep. Parry & Wehr (1987) found that similar sleep deprivation also improved mood in 8 out of 10 women with premenstrual depression, with improvement sustained beyond the night of recovery sleep.

### (ii) Neurotransmitter receptor levels in the peripheral blood

There is now substantial evidence to suggest that a decrease in central serotonergic activity increases the vulnerability to depression. Earlier studies reported a decrease in platelet imipramine bindings sites in depressed patients (e.g. Briley *et al.* 1980). However, more recent studies have presented a conflicting picture, probably because of the many methodological problems with this type of assay. Problems in interpreting such evidence in terms of CNS activity was mentioned earlier, though a consistent association between plasma levels and depressive state would be of considerable interest. As yet, however, the measurement of platelet 5-HT receptor levels as a biological marker of depression or the propensity for depression must be regarded as of uncertain value (Cowen & Wood, 1991). The limited evidence from studies of levels of 5-HT and its receptors in the blood, at different stages of the menstrual cycle, in women with and without premenstrual mood change, was summarized earlier.

### (iii) Neuroendocrine challenge tests

Although, as discussed earlier, the mediation of the pituitary response to exogenous endocrine or pharmacological challenges is obviously complex, the response to a specific challenge does provide some information about the functioning of neurotransmitter systems in the hypothalamus. Thus clonidine, an alpha-2 agonist, elicits a growth hormone (GH) response which is blunted in depressive illness and panic disorder (Cowen & Wood, 1991).

The challenge to the serotonergic system which has been most extensively studied is i.v. L-tryptophan, the precursor of 5-HT. The normal prolactin and GH responses to L-tryptophan are blunted in states of depression (Koyama & Meltzer, 1986; Cowen & Charig, 1987; Deakin *et al.* 1990), although the responsiveness can be complicated by dieting and weight loss (Cowen & Anderson, 1991). This blunting is not apparent in panic disorder or obsessional neurosis, suggesting an effect more specific to depression.

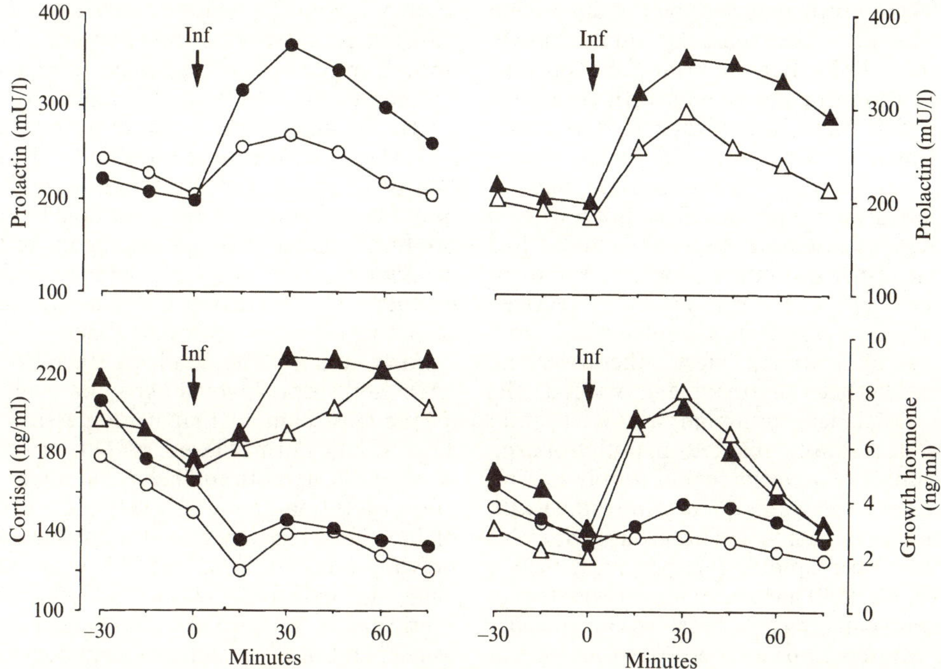



FIG. 4. Endocrine responses to i.v. L-tryptophan challenge in two groups of women, with premenstrual depression (MC group) and without premenstrual depression (NMC group), carried out twice, once in the premenstrual phase and once postmenstrually (○, MC pre; ●, MC post; △, NMC pre; ▲, NMC post). The prolactin response was significantly blunted premenstrually in both groups of women. The cortisol and GH responses were significantly blunted in the MC group *on both occasions*. (From Bancroft *et al.* 1991.)

Also, the responses return to normal after clinical recovery from depression, suggesting a 'state' rather than a 'trait' phenomenon (Upadyhaya *et al.* 1991).

One study of the neuroendocrine response to L-tryptophan in women with premenstrual depression and controls has been reported and was mentioned earlier (Bancroft *et al.* 1991). The prolactin response during the premenstrual phase was blunted in both patients and controls, suggesting that some alteration in 5-HT activity *normally* occurs during the luteal phase but is not sufficient itself to produce negative mood. The GH response and, somewhat unexpectedly, the cortisol response were blunted in the patients *both premenstrually and postmenstrually* (see Fig. 4). It is not clear why the GH response behaved differently, although there may be other factors which more specifically limit the GH response. The cortisol response, as mentioned earlier, is not understood. It was postulated that these effects reflected some form of 'state' vulnerability. The significance of the blunted cortisol response will be considered further below.

In a further study using oral D-fenfluramine as the challenge, women with premenstrual depression showed a blunted prolactin response compared to controls, but both premenstrually and postmenstrually, and neither group showed a cycle phase effect (Bancroft *et al.* 1993*b*). There was also no significant cortisol response in either group. The different 5-HT receptor sub-types implicated in the neuroendocrine responses to L-tryptophan and D-fenfluramine, discussed earlier, may account for these discrepant findings.

The possibility that abnormalities of thyroid function are involved in the causation of PMS has been raised on a number of occasions, with one report, claiming therapeutic benefits of thyroid hormone, attracting considerable publicity (Brayshaw & Brayshaw, 1986). No consistent evidence of hypothyroidism has been found, though a number of studies have assessed the TSH and prolactin response to TRH. This is a further example of a neuroendocrine challenge test associated with a blunted response in depressive illness (Witschy *et al.* 1984). Schmidt *et al.* (1993) recently reported their findings from a series of studies concerning thyroid function in women with PMS. Basal thyroid function tests were carried out in 124 women with confirmed PMS; 10·5% had either Grade I or II hypothyroidism or hyperthyroidism. In 63 women thyroid autoantibodies were assessed and elevated levels were found in 13%. Sixty women had TRH stimulation tests and 30% had abnormal responses; either blunted ($N = 6$) or exaggerated ($N = 12$). Thirty women received thyroxine and placebo in a double-blind cross over study of treatment effects; there were no differences between thyroxine and placebo. The authors concluded 'although it is clear that PMS is not simply masked hypothyroidism, abnormalities of thyroid function appear with greater than expected frequency in women with PMS and may define a sub-group with this disorder'. Other studies (Casper *et al.* 1989; Nikolai *et al.* 1990) have been more consistent in their negative findings. At most we can consider thyroid dysfunction as one possible factor, among others, contributing to 'vulnerability'.

### (iv) The hypophyseal–pituitary–adrenal (HPA) axis

One of the most robust neuroendocrine abnormalities associated with depressive illness is overactivity of the HPA axis, although such changes are not confined to affective disorder. This is manifested as increased levels of circulating cortisol noticeable mainly in the evening when, normally there is a marked circadian decline. There is also, typically, relative resistance to dexamethasone suppression. The ACTH response to corticotrophin releasing hormone (CRH) is blunted, suggesting a high baseline level of CRH and the negative feedback effect of increased circulating cortisol on the pituitary (Orth, 1992). The adrenal cortex appears to be hypersensitive to ACTH stimulation with the increased cortisol production keeping ACTH release in check (Gold *et al.* 1984). CRH levels in CSF are raised in depressive illness (Banki *et al.* 1987) and CRH binding sites are decreased in number in the cerebral cortex of suicide victims, consistent with a down-regulation of receptors resulting from hypersecretion (Nemeroff *et al.* 1988).

While hyperactivity of the HPA axis in depressive illness has been recognized for many years, its functional significance remains unknown. Is it an epiphenomenon of altered neurotransmitter activity in the hypothalamus, or does it represent some adaptive reaction to counteract the effects of the depressed mood? CRH, the neuropeptide mainly responsible for ACTH release, does have other neurotransmitter or neuromodulator effects in extra-hypothalamic brain areas, and its administration to animals produces changes that are analogous to human depression. This has led Nemeroff (1988) to postulate that increased CRH production is a causative factor in depressive illness.

Early attempts to investigate the HPA axis in PMS not surprisingly looked for evidence of overactivity akin to that of depressive illness. They found normal levels of 24 h urinary free cortisol during both follicular and luteal phases of the cycle (Haskett *et al.* 1984) and no evidence of increased resistance to dexamethasone suppression (Haskett *et al.* 1984; Roy-Byrne *et al.* 1986). In one study (Watts *et al.* 1985), significantly higher but normal levels of plasma cortisol were found in PMS sufferers than controls, but in both phases of the cycle.

More recent studies have raised interestingly different possibilities. Rabin *et al.* (1990) studied 7 women with premenstrual mood change and 7 controls. Daily urinary free cortisol measurement was carried out throughout the cycle. Averaging the levels for each half of the cycle showed no difference between groups and none between the follicular and luteal phase. On two occasions, premenstrually (day $24 \pm 3$) and early in the follicular phase (day $5 \pm 3$), and between 18.00 and 21.00 h in the evening, CRH stimulation tests were carried out. The baseline levels from these two tests showed significantly lower plasma cortisol in the PMS women *on both occasions*. ACTH levels did not differ. There was a non-significant tendency for the PMS women to show a greater increase of ACTH in response to the CRH, and a greater increase in cortisol, which was significant when the premenstrual and postmenstrual tests were combined. The greater cortisol response in the PMS group was from a lower baseline, resulting in peak levels which were very similar to those of the controls. Nevertheless, although these differences in HPA activity were subtle, they were in the opposite direction to those expected in depressive illness, and, if anything, suggest *underactivity* of the HPA axis in women with PMS at *both phases of the cycle*. (It should be noted that the follicular test was carried out relatively early in the cycle when some of the PMS women may still have been experiencing negative mood.)

The cortisol response to i.v. L-tryptophan, mentioned earlier (Bancroft *et al.* 1991) is of related interest. This study showed a lack of cortisol response to an L-tryptophan challenge in women with perimenstrual depression, *both premenstrually and postmenstrually*. This led us to speculate that the cortisol response to L-tryptophan, observed in the controls, reflected a reactivity of the HPA axis which was protective against negative mood change otherwise induced during the late luteal phase. Women who, for some reason, are unable to show this HPA reactivity may be more at risk for experiencing perimenstrual depression. The idea that an increase in HPA activity may be protective against depression, while consistent with the role of the axis in stress, may conflict with the common association of overactivity and depressive illness. However, in the case of perimenstrual depression, we are considering mood change at an early stage of its development. It is not known when, in the development of a major depressive illness, the HPA overactivity becomes established. But it may be at a relatively late stage when regulatory mechanisms have become disrupted. Alternatively, as Rabin *et al.* (1990) suggested, there may be two types of disordered function of the HPA axis related to negative mood, one characterized by an enhanced and the other a blunted response to CRH.

Further research into the reactivity of the HPA axis in women with premenstrual depression is clearly warranted. Some form of altered responsiveness of the axis may well contribute to the vulnerability factor.

### B. Autonomic reactivity

The evidence for cycle-related changes in cortical (CNS) arousal and peripheral autonomic reactivity were discussed briefly above. Asso & Magos (1992) studied both these aspects in women with severe PMS as well as controls. In measures of cortical arousal (two flash fusion), which in most studies tends to show a decline premenstrually, the two groups of women did not differ during the follicular phase, but the women with PMS showed a substantially greater premenstrual decline, so that at that stage of the cycle the two groups were significantly different. In terms of autonomic reactivity, measured by

electrodermal activity, patients showed markedly greater responsiveness than the controls at both phases of the cycle, with little change between the two phases in either group. Such differences were not found by Van den Akker & Steptoe (1989).

Thus, while this evidence is still limited, (and with relatively small numbers involved, variation between studies is to be expected), we have some evidence to suggest that central or cortical arousal commonly shows a decline premenstrually which is accentuated in women with premenstrual mood change. Autonomic reactivity, on the other hand, in some women with PMS, appears to be more marked (and of maladaptive significance) *throughout* the cycle, once again suggesting an aspect of vulnerability.

## VIII. THE PLACEBO RESPONSE

A consistent finding in treatment studies of 'PMS' has been a high rate of placebo response, ranging from 40 % (Sampson, 1979) to 94 % (Magos *et al.* 1986 *b*). The nature of this response, its duration, the types of symptoms responding and the distinguishing characteristics of the responder are issues which have received little attention in the PMS literature (Bancroft & Bäckström, 1985). In some studies, improvement in response to placebo has been more marked in mood than in physical symptoms (Sampson, 1979; Metcalf & Hudson, 1985). Other studies have not found this distinction (Maddocks *et al.* 1986; Sampson *et al.* 1988). There are clearly some women who respond to placebo and others who do not. In a study of 31 women, 21 continued to experience PMS, with unchanged severity, in spite of placebo treatment; 8 women, who previously had shown a consistent PMS pattern, lost it with placebo treatment (Metcalf & Hudson, 1985). Harrison *et al.* (1984) compared placebo responders and non-responders; the only significant difference was that the non-responders were more likely to have sought treatment for PMS previously.

'PMS' is not unusual as a clinical problem in showing a substantial likelihood of response to placebo. Unfortunately, however, the extent of this response is often taken to mean that the complaints themselves are not 'serious' or 'real', or not worthy of scientific study. Placebo response is central to much of medical care and we are still remarkably ignorant about the underlying mechanisms. It has been postulated that conditioning is the basic mediating mechanism (Turkkan & Brady, 1985). Such explanations are plausible in some circumstances but not all. Biological mechanisms have also been considered; there is evidence, based on the experimental use of opioid antagonists, that placebo relief of pain is mediated by endogenous opioid release (Grevert & Goldstein, 1985).

A variety of mechanisms may contribute to improvement observed in treatment situations (Bancroft & Bäckström, 1985). Although we have little evidence of the natural history of PMS, it is likely that many women experience worsening of their typical cycle-related changes over a number of months. In such circumstances, it would not be surprising if a recent phase had already passed its peak by the time the sufferer obtained medical help. The effect of having a clinician take one's problems seriously may sufficiently improve one's self-esteem that symptoms are better tolerated. The simple expectation that help is imminent may reduce distress. The process of monitoring symptoms, now widely used as part of clinical assessment in addition to its use in treatment outcome studies, may have beneficial effects.

Nevertheless, the placebo response remains of crucial importance to our understanding of menstrual cycle-related problems and deserves much closer scrutiny from researchers.

## IX. CONCLUSIONS

The evidence relating perimenstrual symptoms to the ovarian cycle suggests that whereas ovulation *per se* may not be playing a crucial part, cyclic variation of ovarian steroids probably is; stabilizing ovarian steroid levels is quite likely to reduce the intensity of cycle-related symptoms. However, we remain uncertain whether this relationship between varying levels of ovarian steroids and mood-related CNS activity depends upon a direct effect of steroids on brain function or, rather differently, reflects a biological time-keeping role for the ovary, entraining an inherent rhythmicity of CNS function. The evidence for this latter explanation is as yet very limited, but is sufficiently tantalizing to warrant further research.

Whatever the explanation, it is now clear that the precise temporal relationship between such cyclical symptoms and the menstrual cycle can vary, and may be more variable in relation to some types of cyclical change (e.g. mood) than to others (e.g. breast tenderness). This emphasizes the limitations that may result from imposing some arbitrary and relatively inflexible definition of what constitutes a cyclical pattern, and even more so a cyclical 'syndrome'. This review has aimed to demonstrate the extent to which the premenstrual syndrome has become a social rather than a scientific construct, and to convince the reader of the need to break away from such restrictive ways of thinking.

Towards this end, a reformulation of menstrual cycle problems has been suggested, and the relevant evidence re-appraised according to the revised agenda that results. The 'three factor' model proposed should be regarded as a first step towards 'deconstructing' the PMS concept and re-organizing our thinking. It is clearly a simplistic model, but one which does lend itself to elaboration and development.

It should not be assumed, for example, that these three factors represent independent influences. If there is a tendency for 5-HT activity to be impaired in the mood-regulating centres of the brain during the late luteal phase, and if one manifestation of the propensity for suffering depressive illness is also a tendency to underactivity in this serotonergic system, then we should not be surprised to find women with such a depressive tendency also prone to premenstrual mood change, and of a somewhat prolonged variety. It remains a possibility that factors involved in the build-up to menstruation may in some way accentuate or aggravate these neurotransmitter changes. The 'timing factor', as we have called it, may vary in its impact from woman to woman, even though such effects may be of minor clinical significance.

However, there are many obvious advantages of this three-factor approach. First, it allows us to defuse the political implications of PMS – in particular the idea that severe PMS is at one end of a continuum of menstrual cycle-related change, implying that such disturbance, whether severe or not, is an essential part of being a woman. Instead we can see that the likelihood of menstrual cycle changes being seriously disruptive is dependent on other factors such as vulnerability, and that in the non-vulnerable woman, cyclical changes are of no consequence, and in fact include a tendency to feel or perform better at certain times, as well as less well at others. It then becomes much easier to see the vulnerability as something which is just as likely to affect men as women.

We can also approach our future research with a fresh agenda. The timing factor, as already mentioned, raises the question of whether we are dealing with direct hormonal influences on the brain, or in a more limited sense, with a biological time keeper. The possibilities raised by the findings of Schmidt *et al.* (1991) and McNeill (1992) should lead to many fascinating research studies on this issue. The question of whether there is a cyclical variation in neurotransmitter activity in the CNS linked to the ovarian cycle also becomes a central issue. In our attempts to answer this question, we should have realistic expectations. We are not going to be able to investigate directly varying neurotransmitter activity in specific brain areas of women. However, methods of 'challenging' the *system* offer interesting possibilities, as long as we are not misled by incorrect interpretation of the mediating processes. The possibility of a pituitary factor accounting for varying prolactin responses was discussed as an example of this. Also, the degree of variation in endocrine parameters (e.g. oestradiol) during the cycle may indicate that testing on only two occasions in the cycle is not sufficient.

There are obvious advantages in testing the system in ways which are of more direct relevance to our subject i.e. the mood and well-being of the subject. Thus, measurement of the sedation caused by a clonidine challenge may be more relevant than the neuroendocrine response to it. Similarly, with the serotonergic system, the measurement of the effects of acute tryptophan depletion on mood at different stages of the cycle offers some exciting possibilities which have not yet been explored (Young *et al.* 1988). The oral contraceptive regime, and its manipulation, and the LHRH analogues also offer rich opportunities. Particular attention has been drawn to food craving, as a possible marker of the 'timing factor'. This looks like a promising approach, but there is much to be done before we will be able to understand the relevance of this common phenomenon to perimenstrual mood changes. Clumsiness is another common phenomenon which may be directly related to the 'timing factor' but which has been largely ignored. Compared with many menstrual cycle complaints, this lends itself to objective methods of assessment.

When we consider the 'menstruation factor' we are confronted with the contrast between 'menstrual relief', a phenomenon which remains ill understood, and 'menstrual aggravation', a less surprising effect even though its precise mechanisms have not yet been identified. Metcalf's group has shown us how fruitful the comparison can be of women with and without a uterus. This model deserves further exploration. The psychological factors associated with menorrhagia have also been seriously neglected, in spite of widespread recognition that a substantial proportion of women who complain of menorrhagia are in fact losing acceptable amounts of blood. Similarly, the relationship between pain, particularly that experienced during the premenstrual phase, and mood, deserves closer scrutiny.

Finally, the 'vulnerability factor' confronts us with a wide range of clinically relevant issues, which can be conceptualized in both psychosocial and biological terms. It will probably be possible to demonstrate that vulnerability, in this sense, is the most crucial clinical issue in attempting to help women suffering with menstrual cycle-related problems. This recognition is not necessarily going to make it easier to help such women, but it may result in a clearer idea of what the needs for help are.

Many of the previously puzzling aspects of PMS become less puzzling when the 'vulnerability' factor is taken into account. The considerable variation, in intensity as well as timing, of symptoms from one cycle to another, which characterizes a large proportion of the women that attend PMS clinics, has always been difficult to explain in terms of ovarian dysfunction. Variation in vulnerability, on the other hand, is much less difficult to comprehend, particularly when we see vulnerability as a 'state' issue. Similarly, the placebo response becomes easier to understand, although the characteristics of the placebo responder and non-responder still await clarification.

There are many puzzles that will remain, but perhaps now the way ahead looks less perplexing than before.

# REFERENCES

Abel, M. H. (1985). Prostaglandins and leukotrienes in menstruation. *Prostaglandin Perspectives* **1**, 1–4.

Abplanalp, J. M., Livingston, L., Rose, R. M. & Sandwisch, D. (1977). Cortisol and growth hormone responses to psychological stress during the menstrual cycle. *Psychosomatic Medicine* **39**, 158–177.

Adamopoulos, D. A., Loraine, J. A., Lunn, S. F., Coppen, A. & Daly, R. (1972). Endocrine profiles in premenstrual tension. *Clinical Endocrinology* **1**, 283–292.

Andersen, A. N., Larsen, J. F., Streenstrup, O. R., Svendstrup, B. & Nielsen, J. (1977). Effect of bromocriptine on the premenstrual syndrome. A double-blind clinical trial. *British Journal of Obstetrics and Gynaecology* **84**, 370–374.

Anderson, I. M. (1989). Serotonin receptors, buspirone and the premenstrual syndrome. *Lancet* ii, 615.

Ashby, R. C., Jr, Carr, L. A., Cook, C. L. & Steptoe, M. H. (1988). Alteration of platelet serotonergic mechanisms and monoamine oxidase activity in premenstrual syndrome. *Biological Psychiatry* **24**, 225–233.

Asso, D. (1983). *The Real Menstrual Cycle.* Wiley: Chichester.

Asso, D. (1988). Physiology and psychology of the normal menstrual cycle. In *Functional Disorders of the Menstrual Cycle* (ed. M. G. Brush), pp. 15–36. Wiley: Chichester.

Asso, D. & Magos, A. L. (1992). Psychological and physiological changes in severe premenstrual syndrome. *Biological Psychology* **33**, 115–132.

AuBuchon, P. G. & Calhoun, K. S. (1985). Menstrual cycle symptomatology: the role of social expectancy and experimental demand characteristics. *Psychosomatic Medicine* **47**, 35–45.

Ayers, J. W. T. & Gidwani, G. P. (1983). The 'luteal breast': hormonal and sonographic investigation of benign breast disease in patients with cyclic mastalgia. *Fertility and Sterility* **40**, 779–784.

Bäckström, C. T., Boyle, H. & Baird, D. T. (1981). Persistence of symptoms of premenstrual tension in hysterectomised women. *British Journal of Obstetrics and Gynaecology* **88**, 530–536.

Bäckström, T., Sanders, D., Leask, R., Davidson, D., Warner, P. & Bancroft, J. (1983). Mood, sexuality, hormones and the menstrual cycle. II. Hormone levels and their relationship to the premenstrual syndrome. *Psychosomatic Medicine* **45**, 503–507.

Bancroft, J. & Bäckström, T. (1985). Premenstrual syndrome. *Clinical Endocrinology* **22**, 313–336.

Bancroft, J. & Rennie, D. (1993). The impact of oral contraceptives on the experience of perimenstrual mood, clumsiness, food craving and other symptoms. *Journal of Psychosomatic Research* **37**, 195–202.

Bancroft, J. & Sartorius, N. (1990). The effects of oral contraceptives on wellbeing and sexuality. *Oxford Reviews of Reproductive Biology* **12**, 57–92.

Bancroft, J., Boyle, H., Davidson, D. W., Gray, J. & Fraser, H. M. (1985). The effects of an LHRH-analogue on the premenstrual syndrome: a preliminary report. In *LHRH and its Analogues: Fertility and Antifertility Aspects* (ed. M. Schmidt-Gollwitzer and R. Schley), pp. 307–319. Walter De Gruyter & Co.: Berlin.

Bancroft, J., Sanders, D., Warner, P. & Loudon, N. (1987a). The effects of oral contraceptives on mood and sexuality: a comparison of triphasic and combined preparations. *Journal of Psychosomatic Obstetrics and Gynaecology* **7**, 1–8

Bancroft, J., Boyle, H., Warner, P. & Fraser, H. (1987b). The use of an LHRH agonist – buserelin, the long term management of premenstrual syndromes. *Clinical Endocrinology* **27**, 171–182.

Bancroft, J., Boyle, H. & Fraser, H. M. (1987c). An LHRH agonist, administered by nasal spray, as a long term treatment for premenstrual syndrome. An exploratory study. *British Journal of Clinical Practice* **41**, suppl. 48, 53–58.

Bancroft, J., Cook, A. & Williamson, L. (1988). Food craving, mood and the menstrual cycle. *Psychological Medicine* **18**, 855–860.

Bancroft, J., Cook, A., Davidson, D., Bennie, J. & Goodwin, G. (1991). Blunting of neuroendocrine responses to infusion of L-tryptophan in women with perimenstrual mood change. *Psychological Medicine* **21**, 305–312.

Bancroft, J., Williamson, L., Warner, P., Rennie, D. & Smith, S. (1993a). Perimenstrual complaints in women complaining of PMS, menorrhagia and dysmenorrhoea: towards a dismantling of the premenstrual syndrome. *Psychosomatic Medicine* **55**, 133–145.

Bancroft, J., Cook, A. & Cooper, I. (1993b). Blunting of neuroendocrine response to D-fenfluramine in women with perimenstrual mood change. Submitted for publication.

Bancroft, J., Rennie, D. & Warner, P. (1993c). Vulnerability to perimenstrual mood change; the relevance of a past history of depressive disorder. *Psychosomatic Medicine* (in the press).

Banki, C. M., Bissette, G., Arato, M., O'Connor, L. & Nemeroff, C. B. (1987). CSF corticotrophin-releasing factor-like immunoreactivity in depression and schizophrenia. *American Journal of Psychiatry* **144**, 873–877.

Barbieri, R. L. & Ryan, J. R. (1981). Danazol: endocrine pharmacology and therapeutic applications. *American Journal of Obstetrics and Gynecology* **141**, 453–463.

Baron, M., Levitt, M. & Periman, R. (1980). Human platelet monoamine oxidase and the menstrual cycle. *Psychiatry Research* **3**, 323–327.

Belmaker, R. H., Murphy, D. L., Wyatt, R. J. & Loriaux, L. (1974). Human platelet monoamine oxidase changes during the menstrual cycle. *Archives of General Psychiatry* **31**, 553–556.

Best, N. R., Rees, M. P., Barlow, D. H. & Cowen, P. J. (1992). Effect of oestradiol treatment on 5-HT and dopamine-mediated neuroendocrine responses. *Journal of Psychopharmacology* **6**, 483–488.

Biegon, A., Bercovitz, H. & Samuel, D. (1980). Serotonin receptor concentration during the oestrous cycle of the rat. *Brain Research* **187**, 221–225.

Blundell, J. E. & Hill, A. J. (1989). Effect of D-fenfluramine on appetite in lean and obese human subjects and on changes associated with PMS (premenstrual syndrome). In *Serotonin, from Cell Biology to Pharmacology and Therapeutics* (ed. R. Paoletti and P. M. Vanhoutte), pp. 645–649. Kluwer Academic Publishers: Amsterdam.

Both-Orthman, B., Rubinow, D. R., Hoban, M. C., Malley, J. & Grover, G. N. (1988). Menstrual cycle phase-related changes in appetite in patients with premenstrual syndrome and in control subjects. *American Journal of Psychiatry* **145**, 628–631.

Bowen, D. J. & Grunberg, N. E. (1990). Variations in food preference and consumption across the menstrual cycle. *Physiology and Behavior* **47**, 287–291.

Boyd, A. E. & Sanchez-Franco, E. (1976). Changes in prolactin response to thyrotrophin releasing hormone during the menstrual cycle of normal women. *Journal of Clinical Endocrinology and Metabolism* **44**, 985–989.

Brayshaw, N. D. & Brayshaw, D. D. (1986). Premenstrual syndrome and thyroid function. *Integrative Psychiatry* **5**, 179–193.

Brenner, R. M. & Maslar, I. A. (1988). The primate oviduct and endometrium. In *Physiology of Reproduction*, vol. I (ed. E. Knobil and J. D. Neill), pp. 303–329. Raven Press: New York.

Briley, M. S. R., Langer, S. Z., Raisman, R., Sechter, D. & Zarifian, E. (1980). Tritiated imipramine binding sites are decreased in platelets of untreated depressed patients. *Science* **209**, 303–305.

Brzezinski, A. A., Wurtman, J. J., Wurtman, R. J., Gleason, R., Greenfield, J. & Nader, T. (1990). D-Fenfluramine suppresses the increased calorie and carbohydrate intake and improves the mood of women with premenstrual depression. *Obstetrics and Gynecology* **76**, 296–301.

Buckman, M., Peake, G. T. & Srivastava, L. S. (1976). Endogenous oestrogen modulates phenothiazine-stimulated prolactin secretion. *Journal of Clinical Endocrinology and Metabolism* **43**, 901–906.

Casper, R. F., Patel-Christopher, A. & Powell, A. M. (1989). Thyrotrophin and prolactin responses to thyrotrophin-releasing hormone in premenstrual syndrome. *Journal of Clinical Endocrinology and Metabolism* **68**, 608–612.

Casper, R. F. & Hearn, M. T. (1990). The effect of hysterectomy and bilateral oophorectomy in women with severe premenstrual syndrome. *American Journal of Obstetrics and Gynecology* **162**, 105–109.

Casson, P., Hahn, P. M., Van Vugt, D. A. & Reid, R. L. (1990). Lasting response to ovariectomy in severe intractable premenstrual syndrome. *American Journal of Obstetrics and Gynecology* **162**, 99–105.

Cawood, E., Bancroft, J. & Steel, J. M. (1993). Perimenstrual symptoms in women with diabetes mellitus and their relationship to diabetic control. *Diabetic Medicine* **10**, 444–448.

Cohen, I. T., Sherwin, B. B. & Fleming, A. S. (1987). Food cravings, mood and the menstrual cycle. *Hormones and Behavior* **21**, 457–470.

Collins, A., Eneroth, P. & Landgren, B. (1985). Psychoneuroendocrine stress responses and mood as related to the menstrual cycle. *Psychosomatic Medicine* **47**, 512–527.

Coppen, A. & Kessel, N. (1963). Menstruation and personality. *British Journal of Psychiatry* **109**, 711–721.

Coppen, A. J., Milne, H. B., Outram, D. H. & Weber, J. C. P. (1969). Dytide, norethisterone and a placebo in the premenstrual syndrome. A double blind comparison. *Clinical Trials Journal* **6**, 33–35.

Costello, C. G. (1992). Research on symptoms versus research on syndromes. Arguments in favour of allocating more research time to the study of symptoms. *British Journal of Psychiatry* **160**, 304–308.

Cowen, P. J. (1992). Neuroendocrine measures of 5-HT receptor subtype function in depression. In *Advances in the Biosciences* (ed. P. B. Bradley, S. L. Handley, S. J. Cooper, B. J. Key, N. M. Barnes and J. H. Coote), pp. 287–296. Pergamon Press: New York.

Cowen, P. J. & Charig, E. M. (1987). Neuroendocrine responses to intravenous tryptophan in major depression. *Archives of General Psychiatry* **44**, 958–966.

Cowen, P. J. & Anderson, I. M. (1991). Abnormal 5-HT neuroendocrine function in depression: association or artefact? In *5-Hydroxytryptamine in Psychiatry: A Spectrum of Ideas* (ed. M. Sandler, A. Coppen and S. Harnett), pp. 121–145. Oxford University Press: Oxford.

Cowen, P. J. & Wood, A. J. (1991). Biological markers of depression. *Psychological Medicine* **21**, 831–836.

Craig, G. (1980). The premenstrual syndrome and prostaglandin metabolism. *British Journal of Family Planning* **6**, 74–77.

Cullberg, J. (1972). Mood changes and menstrual symptoms with different gestagen/estrogen combinations. A double blind comparison with placebo. *Acta Psychiatrica Scandinavica* **Suppl. 236**, 1–86.

*DSM-III-R*, (1987). Appendix A: Proposed diagnostic categories needing further study. pp. 367–369. APA: Washington, DC.

Dalton, K. (1984): *Premenstrual Syndrome and Progesterone Therapy*. Heinemann: London.

Dalton, K. & Holton, W. M. (1992). Diet of women with severe premenstrual syndrome and the effect of changing to a three-hourly starch diet. *Stress Medicine* **8**, 61–65.

Dalvit, S. P. (1981). The effect of the menstrual cycle on patterns of food intake. *American Journal of Clinical Nutrition* **34**, 1811–1815.

Dalvit-McPhillips, S. P. (1983). The effect of the human menstrual cycle on nutrient intake. *Physiology and Behavior* **31**, 209–212.

Day, J. (1979). Danazol and the premenstrual syndrome. *Postgraduate Medicine* **55**, Suppl. 5, 87–89.

DeJong, R., Rubinow, D. R., Roy-Byrne, P., Hoban, M. C., Grover, G. N. & Post, R. M. (1985). Premenstrual mood disorder and psychiatric illness. *American Journal of Psychiatry* **142**, 1359–1361.

Deakin, J. F. W., Pennell, I., Upadhyaya, A. J. & Lofthouse, R. (1990). A neuroendocrine study of 5HT function in depression: evidence for biological mechanisms of endogenous and psychosocial causation. *Psychopharmacology* **101**, 85–92.

Dennerstein, L., Spencer-Gardiner, C. & Brown, J. B. (1984). Premenstrual tension: hormonal profiles. *Journal of Psychosomatic Obstetrics and Gynaecology* **3**, 37–51.

Dennerstein, L., Spencer-Gardner, C., Gotts, G., Brown, J. B., Smith, M. A. & Burrows, G. D. (1985). Progesterone and the premenstrual syndrome: a double blind crossover trial. *British Medical Journal* **290**, 1617–1621.

Dinan, T. G., Barry, S., Yatham, L. N., Mobayed, M. & O'Hanlon, M. (1990). The reproducibility of the prolactin response to buspirone: relationship to the menstrual cycle. *International Clinical Psychopharmacology* **5**, 119–123.

Dye, L. (1992). Psychophysical measures of visual information processing. In *Cognition and the Menstrual Cycle* (ed. J. T. E. Richardson), pp. 67–97. Springer: New York.

Eckerd, M. B., Hurt, S. W. & Severino, S. K. (1989). Late luteal phase dysphoric disorder: relationship to personality disorders. *Journal of Personality Disorders* **4**, 338–344.

Endicott, J., Halbreich, U., Schacht, S. & Nee, J. (1985). Affective disorder and premenstrual depression. In *Premenstrual Syndrome: Current Findings and Future Directions* (ed. H. J. Osofsky and S. J. Blumenthal), pp. 3–11. American Psychiatric Press: Washington, DC.

Englander-Golden, P., Whitmore, M. R. & Dienstbier, R. A. (1978). Menstrual cycle as focus of study and self-reports of moods and behaviors. *Motivation and Emotion* **2**, 75–86.

Faratian, B., Gaspar, A., O'Brien, P. M. S., Johnson, I. R., Filshie, G. M. & Prescott, P. (1984). Premenstrual syndrome: weight, abdominal swelling, and perceived body image. *American Journal of Obstetrics and Gynecology* **150**, 200–204.

Fernstrom, J. D. & Wurtman, R. J. (1971). Brain serotonin content: increase following ingestion of carbohydrate diet. *Science* **174**, 1023–1025.

Fernstrom, J. D. & Wurtman, R. J. (1972). Brain serotonin content: physiological regulation by plasma neutral amino acids. *Science* **178**, 414–416.

Fradkin, B. & Firestone, P. (1986). Premenstrual tension, expectancy, and mother–child relations. *Journal of Behavioral Medicine* **9**, 245–259.

Freeman, E. W., Sondheimer, S., Weinbaum, P. J. & Rickels, K. (1985). Evaluating premenstrual symptoms in medical practice. *Obstetrics and Gynecology* **65**, 500–505.

Gallant, S. J., Popiel, D. A., Hoffman, D. M., Chakraborty, P. K. & Hamilton, J. A. (1992). Using daily ratings to confirm premenstrual syndrome/late luteal phase dysphoric disorder. Part 1. Effects of demand characteristics and expectations. *Psychosomatic Medicine* **54**, 149–166.

Gold, P. W., Chrousos, G., Kellner, C., Post, R., Augerinos, P., Schulte, H., Oldfield, E. & Loriaux, D. L. (1984). Psychiatric implications of basic and clinical studies with corticotrophin-releasing factor. *American Journal of Psychiatry* **141**, 619–627.

Goldberg, D. P. & Huxley, P. (1991). *Common Mental Disorders: A Biosocial Model*. Routledge: London.

Graham, C. A. & Sherwin, B. B. (1987). The relationship between retrospective premenstrual symptom reporting and present oral contraceptive use. *Journal of Psychosomatic Research* **31**, 45–53.

Graham, C. A. (1989). Treatment of premenstrual syndrome with a triphasic oral contraceptive: a double blind placebo-controlled study. Ph.D thesis. McGill University, Montreal.

Graham, C. A. & Sherwin, B. B. (1992). A prospective treatment study of premenstrual symptoms using a triphasic oral contraceptive. *Journal of Psychosomatic Research* **36**, 257–266.

Grant, E. C. G. & Pryse-Davies, J. (1968). Effect of oral contraceptives on depressive mood changes and on endometrial monoamine oxidase and phosphatase. *British Medical Journal* **iii**, 777–780.

Grevert, P. & Goldstein, A. (1985). Placebo analgesia, naloxone, and the role of endogenous opioids. In *Placebo: Theory, Research and*

*Mechanisms* (ed. L. White, B. Tursky and G. E. Schwartz), pp. 332–350. Guilford: New York.

Halbreich, U. & Endicott, J. (1982). Classification of premenstrual syndromes. In *Behaviour and the Menstrual Cycle* (ed. R. C. Friedman), pp. 243–265. Marcel Dekker, Inc.: New York.

Halbreich, U., Endicott, J., Schacht, S. & Nee, J. (1982). The diversity of premenstrual changes as reflected in the Premenstrual Assessment form. *Acta Psychiatrica Scandinavica* 65, 46–65.

Halbreich, U. & Endicott, J. (1985a). Methodological issues in studies of premenstrual changes. *Psychoneuroendocrinology* 10, 15–32.

Halbreich, U. & Endicott, J. (1985b). The relationship of dysphoric premenstrual changes to depressive disorder. *Acta Psychiatrica Scandinavica* 71, 331–338.

Hammarbäck, S., Bäckström, T., Holst, J. V., Schoultz, B. & Lyrenas, S. (1985). Cyclical mood changes as in the premenstrual tension syndrome during sequential estrogen–progestagen post-menopausal replacement therapy. *Acta Obstetricia et Gynecologica Scandinavica* 64, 393–397.

Hammarbäck, S. & Bäckström, T. (1988). Induced anovulation as treatment of premenstrual tension syndrome. *Acta Obstetricia et Gynecologica Scandinavica* 67, 159–166.

Hammarbäck, S. & Bäckström, T. (1989). Cyclical symptoms disappeared during anovulation in PMS. *Journal of Psychosomatic Obstetrics and Gynaecology* 10, Suppl. 1, 157.

Hammarbäck, S., Bäckström, T. & MacGibbon-Taylor, B. (1989). Diagnosis of premenstrual tension syndrome: description and evaluation of a procedure for diagnosis and differential diagnosis. *Journal of Psychosomatic Obstetrics and Gynaecology* 10, 25–42.

Hargrove, J. T. & Abraham, G. E. (1982). The incidence of premenstrual tension in a gynaecologic clinic. *Journal of Reproductive Medicine* 27, 721–724.

Harrison, W. M., Endicott, J., Rabkin, J. G. & Nee, J. (1984). Treatment of premenstrual dysphoric changes: clinical outcome and methodological implications. *Psychopharmacology Bulletin* 20, 118–122.

Hart, W. G., Coleman, G. J. & Russell, J. W. (1987). Assessment of premenstrual symptomatology: a re-evaluation of the predictive validity of self-report. *Journal of Psychosomatic Research* 31, 185–190.

Haskett, R. F., Steiner, M., Osmun, J. N. & Carroll, B. J. (1980). Severe premenstrual tension: delineation of the syndrome. *Biological Psychiatry* 15, 121–139.

Haskett, R. F., Steiner, M. & Carroll, B. J. (1984). A psychoendocrine study of premenstrual tension syndrome. A model for endogenous depression? *Journal of Abnormal Psychology* 6, 191–199.

Hastrup, J. L. & Light, K. C. (1984). Sex differences in cardiovascular stress responses: modulation as a function of menstrual cycle phases. *Journal of Psychosomatic Research* 28, 475–483.

Hein, P. R. (1975). Motility of the nonpregnant uterus. In *Aspects of Obstetrics Today* (ed. T. K. A. B. Eskes), pp. 259–272. Excerpta Medica: Amsterdam.

Herzberg, B. N., Draper, K. C., Johnson, A. L. & Nicol, G. C. (1971). Oral contraceptives, depression, and libido. *British Medical Journal* iii, 495–500.

Hill, A. J., Weaver, C. F. L. & Blundell, J. E. (1991). Food craving, dietary restraint and mood. *Appetite* 17, 187–197.

Hudgens, G. A., Fatkin, L. T., Billingsley, P. A. & Mazurczak, J. (1988). Hand steadiness: effects of sex, menstrual phase, oral contraceptives, practice, and handgun weight. *Human Factors* 30, 51–60.

Hurt, S. W., Schnurr, P. P., Severino, S. K., Freeman, E. W., Gise, L. H., Rivera-Tovar, A. & Steege, J. F. (1992). Late luteal phase dysphoric disorder in 670 women evaluated for premenstrual complaints. *American Journal of Psychiatry* 149, 525–530.

Illingworth, P. J., Reddi, K., Smith, K. & Baird, D. T. (1990). Pharmacological 'rescue' of the corpus luteum results in increased inhibin production. *Clinical Endocrinology* 33, 323–332.

Jakubowicz, D. L., Godard, E. & Dewhurst, J. (1984). The treatment of premenstrual tension with mefenamic acid: analysis of prosta-glandin concentrations. *British Journal of Obstetrics and Gynaecology* 91, 78–84.

Jones, E. M., Fox, R. H., Verow, P. W. & Asscher, A. W. (1966). Variations in capillary permeability to plasma problems during the menstrual cycle. *Journal of Obstetrics and Gynaecology of the British Commonwealth* 73, 666–669.

Jordheim, O. (1972). The premenstrual syndrome. Clinical trials of treatment with a progestagen combined with a diuretic compared with both a progestagen alone and a placebo. *Acta Obstetricia et Gynecologica Scandinavica* 51, 77–80.

Kashiwagi, T., McClure, J. N. & Wetzell, R. D. (1976). Premenstrual affective syndrome and psychiatric disorder. *Diseases of the Nervous System* 37, 116–119.

Kendell, R. E. (1975). *The Role of Diagnosis in Psychiatry*. Blackwell Scientific Publications: Oxford.

Keye, W. R. Jr, Hammond, D. C. & Strang, T. (1986). Medical and psychological characteristics of women presenting with premenstrual symptoms. *Obstetrics and Gynecology* 68, 634–637.

Koyama, T. & Meltzer, H. Y. (1986). A biochemical and neuro-endocrine study of the serotonergic system in depression. In *New Results of Depression Research* (ed. H. Hippius), pp. 169–188. Springer-Verlag: Berlin.

Kuhl, H., Gahn, G., Romberg, G., Marz, W. & Taubert, H. D. (1985). A randomized cross-over comparison of two low-dose oral contraceptives upon hormonal and metabolic parameters. I. Effects upon sexual hormone levels. *Contraception* 31, 583–593.

Kutner, S. J. & Brown, W. L. (1972). Types of oral contraceptives, depression, and premenstrual symptoms. *Journal of Nervous and Mental Disease* 155, 153–162.

Leinster, S. J., Whitehouse, G. H. & Walsh, P. V. (1987). Cyclical mastalgia: clinical and mammographic observations in a screened population. *British Journal of Surgery* 74, 220–222.

Luine, V. N. & McEwen, B. S. (1985). Steroid hormone receptors in brain and pituitary: topography and possible functions. In *Handbook of Behavioral Neurobiology, Volume 7. Reproduction* (ed. N. Adler, D. Pfaff and R. W. Goy), pp. 665–724. Plenum: New York.

MacDonald, P. C., Dombroski, R. A. & Casey, M. L. (1991). Recurrent secretion of progesterone in large amounts: an endocrine/metabolic disorder unique to young women? *Endocrine Reviews* 12, 372–400.

Mackenzie, T. B., Wilcox, K. & Baron, H. (1986). Lifetime prevalence of psychiatric disorders in women with perimenstrual difficulties. *Journal of Affective Disorders* 10, 15–19.

McNeill, E. (1992). Variation in subjective state over the oral contraceptive cycle: the influence of endogenous steroids and temporal manipulation. Ph.D. thesis, University of Edinburgh.

McNeilly, A. S. & Hagen, C. (1974). Prolactin, TSH, LH and FSH responses to a combined LHRH/TRH test at different stages of the menstrual cycle. *Clinical Endocrinology* 3, 427–435.

Maddocks, S., Hahn, P., Moller, F. & Reid, R. L. (1986). A double-blind placebo-controlled trial of progesterone vaginal suppositories in the treatment of premenstrual syndrome. *American Journal of Obstetrics and Gynecology* 154, 573–581.

Magos, A. L. & Studd, J. W. W. (1984). The premenstrual syndrome. In *Progress in Obstetrics and Gynaecology* (ed. J. W. W. Studd), pp. 334–350. Churchill Livingstone: Edinburgh.

Magos, A. L., Collins, W. P. & Studd, J. W. W. (1984). Management of the premenstrual syndrome by subcutaneous implants of oestradiol. *Journal of Psychosomatic Obstetrics and Gynaecology* 3, 93–99.

Magos, A. L., Brincat, M. & Studd, J. W. W. (1986a). Trend analysis of the symptoms of 150 women with a history of the premenstrual syndrome. *American Journal of Obstetrics and Gynecology* 155, 277–282.

Magos, A. L., Brincat, M. & Studd, J. W. W. (1986b). Treatment of the premenstrual syndrome by subcutaneous oestradiol implants and cyclical oral norethisterone: placebo controlled study. *British Medical Journal* 292, 1629–1633.

Magos, A. L., Brewster, E., Singh, R., O'Dowd, T., Brincat, M. & Studd, J. W. W. (1986c). The effects of norethisterone in post-menopausal women on oestrogen replacement therapy: a model for the premenstrual syndrome. *British Journal of Obstetrics and Gynaecology* **93**, 1290–1296.

Magyar, D. M., Boyers, S. P., Marshall, J. R. & Abraham, G. E. (1979). Regular menstrual cycles and premenstrual molimina as indicators of ovulation. *Obstetrics and Gynecology* **53**, 411–414.

Mansel, R. E. (1988). Investigation and treatment of cyclical benign breast disease. In *Functional Disorders of the Menstrual Cycle* (ed. M. G. Brush and E. M. Goldsmit), pp. 191–198. Chichester: Wiley.

Mansel, R. E., Wisbey, J. R. & Hughes, L. E. (1982). Controlled trial of the antigonadotrophin danazol in painful nodular benign diseases. *Lancet* i, 928–930.

Marinari, K. T., Leshner, A. & Doyle, M. (1976). Menstrual cycle status and adrenocortical reactivity to psychological stress. *Psychoneuroendocrinology* **1**, 213–218.

Markum, R. A. (1976). Assessment of the reliability of and the effect of neutral instructions on the symptom ratings on the Moos Menstrual Distress Questionnaire. *Psychosomatic Medicine* **38**, 163–172.

Marriot, A. & Faragher, E. B. (1986). An assessment of psychological state associated with the menstrual cycle in users of oral contraceptives. *Journal of Psychosomatic Research* **30**, 41–47.

Matussek, N., Ackenheil, M. & Herz, M. (1984). The dependence of the clonidine test on alcohol drinking habits and the menstrual cycle. *Psychoneuroendocrinology* **9**, 173–177.

Metcalf, M. G. (1983). Incidence of ovulation from the menarche to the menopause: observations of 622 subjects. *New Zealand Medical Journal* **96**, 645–648.

Metcalf, M. G. & Hudson, S. M. (1985). The premenstrual syndrome: selection of women for treatment trials. *Journal of Psychosomatic Research* **29**, 631–638.

Metcalf, M. G., Livesey, J. H., Wells, J. E., Braiden, V., Hudson, S. M. & Bamber, L. (1991). Premenstrual syndrome in hysterectomized women: mood and physical symptom cyclicity. *Journal of Psychosomatic Research* **35**, 555–567.

Metcalf, M. G., Braiden, V., Livesey, J. H. & Wells, J. E. (1992). The premenstrual syndrome: amelioration of symptoms after hysterectomy. *Journal of Psychosomatic Research* **36**, 569–584.

Milligan, D., Drife, J. O. & Short, R. V. (1975). Changes in breast volume during normal menstrual cycles and after oral contraception. *British Medical Journal* iv, 494–496.

Mira, M., Vizzard, J. & Abraham, S. (1985). Personality characteristics in the menstrual cycle. *Journal of Psychosomatic Obstetrics and Gynaecology* **4**, 329–334.

Mira, M., McNeill, D., Fraser, I. S., Vizzard, J. & Abraham, S. (1986). Mefenamic acid in the treatment of premenstrual syndrome. *Obstetrics and Gynecology* **68**, 395–398.

Moos, R. (1969). Assessment of psychological concomitants of oral contraceptives. In *Metabolic Effects of Gonadal Hormones and Contraceptive Steroids* (ed. K. A. Salhanik), pp. 676–705. Plenum: New York.

Moos, R. H. (1968). Psychological aspects of new contraceptives. *Archives of General Psychiatry* **19**, 87–94.

Morris, N. M. & Udry, J. R. (1972). Contraceptive pills and day-by-day feelings of wellbeing. *American Journal of Obstetrics and Gynecology* **113**, 763–765.

Morse, C. A. & Dennerstein, L. (1988). Cognitive therapy for premenstrual syndrome. In *Functional Disorders of the Menstrual Cycle* (ed. M. G. Brush and E. M. Goldsmit), pp. 177–190. Wiley: Chichester.

Mortola, J. F., Girton, L. & Fischer, U. (1991). Successful treatment of severe premenstrual syndrome by combined use of gonadotropin-releasing hormone agonist and estrogen/progestin. *Journal of Clinical Endocrinology and Metabolism* **71**, 252A–F.

Muse, K. N., Cetel, N. S., Futterman, L. A. & Yen, S. S. C. (1984). The premenstrual syndrome. Effects of 'medical ovariectomy'. *New England Journal of Medicine* **311**, 1345–1349.

NIMH National Institute of Mental Health, (1983). Premenstrual Syndrome Workshop. Rockville, MD, April 14–15.

Nemeroff, C. B. (1988). The role of corticotropin-releasing factor in the pathogenesis of major depression. *Pharmacopsychiatry* **21**, 76–82.

Nemeroff, C. B., Owens, M. J., Bissette, G., Andorn, A. C. & Stanley, M. (1988). Reduced corticotropin releasing factor binding sites in the frontal cortex of suicide victims. *Archives of General Psychiatry* **45**, 577–580.

Nikolai, T. F., Mulligan, G. M., Gribble, R. K., Harkins, P. G., Meier, P. R. & Roberts, R. C. (1990). Thyroid function and treatment in premenstrual syndrome. *Journal of Clinical Endocrinology and Metabolism* **70**, 1108–1113.

O'Keane, V., O'Hanlon, M., Webb, M. & Dinan, T. (1991). D-Fenfluramine/prolactin response throughout the menstrual cycle: evidence for an oestrogen-induced alteration. *Clinical Endocrinology* **34**, 289–292.

Oian, P., Tollan, A., Fadnes, H. O., Noddeland, H. & Maltau, J. M. (1987). Transcapillary fluid dynamics during the menstrual cycle. *American Journal of Obstetrics and Gynecology* **156**, 952–957.

Olasov, B. & Jackson, J. (1987). Effects of expectancies on women's reports of moods during the menstrual cycle. *Psychosomatic Medicine* **49**, 65–78.

Orth, D. N. (1992). Corticotropin-releasing hormone in humans. *Endocrine Reviews* **13**, 164–191.

Osborn, M. F. & Gath, D. H. (1990). Psychological and physical determinants of premenstrual symptoms before and after hysterectomy. *Psychological Medicine* **20**, 565–572.

Parlee, M. B. (1974). Stereotypic beliefs about menstruation: a methodological note on the Moos Menstrual Distress Questionnaire and some new data. *Psychosomatic Medicine* **36**, 229–241.

Parlee, M. B. (1982). Changes in moods and activation levels during the menstrual cycle in experimentally naive subjects. *Psychology of Women Quarterly* **72**, 119–131.

Parry, B. L. & Wehr, T. A. (1987). Therapeutic effect of sleep deprivation in patients with premenstrual syndrome. *American Journal of Psychiatry* **144**, 808–810.

Parry, B. L. Mendelson, W. B., Duncan, W. C., Sack, D. A. & Wehr, T. A. (1989). Longitudinal sleep EEG, temperature, and activity measurements across the menstrual cycle in patients with premenstrual depression and in age-matched controls. *Psychiatry Research* **30**, 285–303.

Parry, B. L. Berga, S. L., Kripke, D. F., Klauber, M. R., Laughlin, G. A., Yet, S. C. & Gillin, J. C. (1990). Altered waveform of plasma nocturnal melatonin secretion in premenstrual depression. *Archives of General Psychiatry* **47**, 1139–1146.

Peters, J. R., Elliott, J. & Grahame-Smith, D. G. (1979). Effect of oral contraceptives on platelet noradrenaline and 5-hydroxytryptamine receptors and aggregation. *Lancet* ii, 933–936.

Pilner, P. & Fleming, A. S. (1983). Food intake, body weight, and sweetness preferences over the menstrual cycle in humans. *Physiology and Behavior* **30**, 663–666.

Plante, T. G. & Denney, D. R. (1984). Stress responsivity among dysmenorrheic women at different phases of their menstrual cycle: more ado about nothing. *Behaviour Research and Therapy* **22**, 249–258.

Poirier, M., Benkelfat, C., Galzin, A. & Langer, S. Z. (1986). Platelet H-imipramine binding and steroid hormone serum concentrations during the menstrual cycle. *Psychopharmacology* **88**, 86–89.

Poirier, M. F., Loo, H., Dennis, T., Le Fur, G. & Scatton, B. (1985). Platelet monoamine oxidase activity and plasma 3,4-dihydroxyphenylethylene glycol levels during the menstrual cycle. *Neuropsychobiology* **14**, 165–169.

Rabin, D. S., Schmidt, P. J., Campbell, G., Gold, P. W., Jensvold, M. J., Rubinow, D. R. & Chrousos, G. P. (1990). Hypothalamic-pituitary-adrenal function in patients with the premenstrual syndrome. *Journal of Clinical Endocrinology and Metabolism* **71**, 1158–1162.

Rapkin, A. J., Edelmuth, E., Chang, L. C., Reading, A. E., McGuire, M. & Su, T. (1987). Whole-blood serotonin in premenstrual syndrome. *Obstetrics and Gynecology* **70**, 533–537.

Rausch, J. L. & Janowsky, D. S. (1982). Premenstrual tension: etiology. In *Behaviour and the Menstrual Cycle* (ed. R. C. Friedman), pp. 397–427. Marcel Dekker: New York.

Reid, R. L. (1985). Premenstrual syndrome. *Current Problems in Obstetrics, Gynecology and Fertility* **8**, 1–57.

Reid, R. L. (1986). Premenstrual syndrome: a time for introspection. *American Journal of Obstetrics and Gynecology* **155**, 921–926.

Reid, R. L. & Yen, S. S. C. (1981). Premenstrual syndrome. *American Journal of Obstetrics and Gynecology* **139**, 85–104.

Rogers, M. L. & Harding, S. S. (1981). Retrospective and daily menstrual distress measures in men and women using Moos's instruments (Forms A and T) and modified versions of Moos's instruments. In *The Menstrual Cycle. Vol. 2. Research and Implications for Women's Health* (ed. P. Komnenich, M. McSweeney, J. A. Noak and N. Elder), pp. 71–81. Springer: New York.

Rosenthal, N. E., Cenhart, M., Cabellero, B., Jacobson, F. M., Skwerer, R., Wurtman, J. & Spring, B. (1986). Carbohydrate craving in seasonal affective disorder. Paper presented at the Annual Meeting of the American Psychological Society, Washington, DC.

Roy-Byrne, P. P., Rubinow, D. R., Gwirtsman, H. G., Hoban, M. C. & Grover, G. N. (1986). Cortisol response to dexamethasone in women with premenstrual syndrome. *Neuropsychobiology* **16**, 61–63.

Roy-Byrne, P. P., Rubinow, D. T. R., Hoban, M. C., Grover, G. N. & Blank, D. (1987). TSH and prolactin responses to TRH in patients with premenstrual syndrome. *American Journal of Psychiatry* **144**, 480–484.

Rubinow, D. R. (1987). Practical and ethical aspects of pharmacotherapeutic evaluation. In *Premenstrual Syndrome: Ethical and Legal Implications in a Biomedical Perspective* (ed. B. E. Ginsburg and B. F. Carter), pp. 47–64. Plenum: New York.

Rubinow, D. R. & Schmidt, P. J. (1992). Premenstrual syndrome: a review of endocrine studies. *Endocrinologist* **2**, 47–54.

Rubinow, D. R., Hoban, C., Roy-Byrne, P., Grover, G. N. & Post, R. M. (1985). Premenstrual syndromes: past and future research strategies. *Canadian Journal of Psychiatry* **30**, 467–473.

Ruble, D. N. (1977). Premenstrual symptoms: a reinterpretation. *Science* **197**, 291–292.

Sampson, G. A. (1979). Premenstrual syndrome. A double-blind controlled trial of progesterone and placebo. *British Journal of Psychiatry* **135**, 209–215.

Sampson, G. A., Heathcote, P. R. M., Wordsworth, J., Prescott, P. & Hodgson, A. (1988). Premenstrual syndrome: a double-blind cross-over study of treatment with dydrogesterone and placebo. *British Journal of Psychiatry* **153**, 232–235.

Sanders, D., Warner, P. & Bäckström, T. (1983). Mood, sexuality, hormones and the menstrual cycle. I. Changes in mood and physical state: description of subjects and methods. *Psychosomatic Medicine* **45**, 487–501.

Sarno, A. P., Miller, E. J., Jr. & Lundblad, E. G. (1987). Premenstrual syndrome: beneficial effects of periodic, low-dose danazol. *Obstetrics and Gynecology* **70**, 33–36.

Schechter, D., Bachmann, G. A., Vaitukaitis, J., Phillips, D. & Saperstein, D. (1989). Perimenstrual symptoms: time course of symptom intensity in relation to endocrinologically defined segments of the menstrual cycle. *Psychosomatic Medicine* **51**, 173–194.

Schmidt, P. J., Nieman, L., Grover, G. N., Muller, K. L., Merriam, G. R. & Rubinow, D. R. (1991). Lack of effect of induced menses on symptoms in women with premenstrual syndrome. *New England Journal of Medicine* **324**, 1174–1179.

Schmidt, P. J., Grover, G. N., Roy-Byrne, P. P. & Rubinow, D. R. (1993). Thyroid function in women with premenstrual syndrome. *Journal of Clinical Endocrinology and Metabolism* **76**, 671–674.

Schnurr, P. P. (1989). Measuring amount of symptom change in the diagnosis of premenstrual syndrome. *Journal of Consulting and Clinical Psychology* **1**, 277–283.

Sherwin, B. B. (1991). The impact of different doses of estrogen and progestin on mood and sexual behavior in postmenopausal women. *Journal of Clinical Endocrinology and Metabolism* **72**, 336–343.

Siegel, J. M., Johnson, J. H. & Sarason, I. G. (1979). Life changes and menstrual discomfort. *Journal of Human Stress* **5**, 41–46.

Sommer, B. (1992). Cognitive performance and the menstrual cycle. In *Cognition and the Menstrual Cycle* (ed. J. T. E. Richardson), pp. 39–66. Springer-Verlag: New York.

Spring, B., Chiodo, J. & Bowen, D. J. (1987). Carbohydrates, tryptophan and behavior: a methodological review. *Psychological Bulletin* **102**, 234–256.

Steege, J. F., Stout, A. L. & Rupp, S. L. (1985). Relationships among premenstrual symptoms and menstrual cycle characteristics. *Obstetrics and Gynecology* **65**, 398–402.

Stout, A. L., Steege, J. F., Blazer, D. G. & George, L. K. (1986). Comparison of lifetime psychiatric diagnoses in premenstrual syndrome clinic and community samples. *Journal of Nervous and Mental Disease* **174**, 517–522.

Tam, W. Y. K., Chan, M. & Lees, P. H. K. (1985). The menstrual cycle and platelet 5-HT uptake. *Psychosomatic Medicine* **47**, 352–362.

Tan, Y. M., Steele, P. A. & Judd, S. J. (1986). The effect of physiological changes in ovarian steroids on the prolactin response to gonadotrophic releasing factor. *Clinical Endocrinology* **24**, 71–78.

Taylor, D. L., Mathew, R. J., Beng, T. H. & Weimman, M. L. (1984). Serotonin levels and platelet uptake during premenstrual tension. *Neuropsychobiology* **12**, 16–18.

Turkkan, J. S. & Brady, J. V. (1985). Mediational theory of the placebo effect. In *Placebo: Theory, Research and Mechanisms* (ed. L. White, B. Tursky and G. E. Schwartz), pp. 324–331. Guildford: New York.

Ulmsten, U. (1985). Uterine activity and blood flow in normal and dysmenorrheic women. In *Premenstrual Syndrome and Dysmenorrhoea* (ed. M. Y. Dawood, J. L. McGuire and L. M. Demers), pp. 87–102. Urban and Schwarzenberg: Baltimore.

Upadyhaya, A. K., Pennell, I., Cowen, P. J. & Deakin, J. F. W. (1991). Blunted growth hormone and prolactin responses to 1-tryptophan in depression – a state dependent abnormality. *Journal of Affective Disorders* **21**, 213–218.

Ussher, J. M. (1992). The demise of dissent and the rise of cognition in menstrual-cycle research. In *Cognition and the Menstrual Cycle* (ed. J. T. E. Richardson), pp. 132–173. Springer-Verlag: New York.

Van den Akker, O. & Steptoe, A. (1985). The pattern and prevalence of symptoms during the menstrual cycle. *British Journal of Psychiatry* **147**, 164–169.

Van den Akker, O. & Steptoe, A. (1989). Psychophysiological responses in women reporting severe premenstrual symptoms. *Psychosomatic Medicine* **51**, 319–328.

Van der Meer, Y. G., Benedek-Jaszmann, L. J. & Van Loenen, A. V. (1983). Effect of high dose progesterone on the premenstrual syndrome: a double-blind cross-over study. *Journal of Psychosomatic Obstetrics and Gynaecology* **2**, 220–225.

Vergare, M. J. (1987). Premenstrual syndrome: implications for psychiatric practice. In *Premenstrual syndrome: Ethical and Legal Implications in a Biomedical Perspective* (ed. B. E. Ginsburg & B. F. Carter), pp. 215–222. Plenum: New York.

Walker, A. (1987). The relationship between premenstrual symptoms and the ovarian cycle. Ph.D thesis. University of Edinburgh.

Walker, A. & Bancroft, J. (1990). The relationship between premenstrual symptoms and oral contraceptive use: a controlled study. *Psychosomatic Medicine* **52**, 86–96.

Warner, P. & Bancroft, J. (1988). Mood, sexuality, oral contraceptives and the menstrual cycle. *Journal of Psychosomatic Research* **32**, 417–427.

Warner, P. & Bancroft, J. (1990). Factors related to self-reporting of the premenstrual syndrome. *British Journal of Psychiatry* **157**, 249–260.

Warner, P., Bancroft, J., Dixson, A. & Hampson, M. (1991). The relationship between perimenstrual depressive mood and depressive illness. *Journal of Affective Disorders* **23**, 9–23.

Watson, N. R., Studd, J. W. W., Riddle, A. F. & Savvas, M. (1988). Suppression of ovulation by transdermal oestradiol patches. *British Medical Journal* **297**, 900–901.

Watson, N. R., Studd, J. W. W., Savvas, M., Garnett, T. & Baber,

R. J. (1989). Treatment of severe premenstrual syndrome with oestradiol patches and cyclical oral norethisterone. *Lancet* ii, 730–732.

Watts, J. F., Butt, W. R. & Edwards, R. L. (1987). A clinical trial using danazol for the treatment of premenstrual tension. *British Journal of Obstetrics and Gynaecology* **94**, 30–34.

Watts, J. F., Butt, W. R., Edwards, R. L. & Holder, G. (1985). Hormonal studies in women with premenstrual tension. *British Journal of Obstetrics and Gynaecology* **92**, 247–255.

Wehr, T. A., Wirz-Justice, A., Duncan, W., Gillin, J. C. & Goodwin, F. K. (1979). Phase-advance of the circadian sleep–wake cycle as an antidepressant. *Science* **206**, 710–713

West, C. P. (1990). Inhibition of ovulation with oral progestins – effectiveness in premenstrual syndrome. *European Journal of Gynaecology and Reproductive Biology* **34**, 119–128.

Williams, J. G. C., Martin, A. J. & Hulkenberg-Tromp, T. E. M. L. (1983), PMS in four European countries: part 2. A double-blind placebo controlled study of dydrogesterone. *British Journal of Sexual Medicine* **10**, 8–18.

Witschy, J. K., Schlesser, M. A. & Fulton, C. L. (1984). TRH-induced prolactin release is blunted in females with endogenous unipolar major depression. *Psychiatric Research* **12**, 321–331.

Wolff, P. H. (1987). *Development of Behavioral States and Expressions of Emotions in Early Infancy*. University of Chicago Press: Chicago.

Wong, W. H., Freedman, R. I., Levan, N. F., Hyman, C. & Quilligan, E. J. (1972). Changes in the capillary filtration coefficient of cutaneous vessels in women with premenstrual tension. *American Journal of Obstetrics and Gynecology* **114**, 950–955.

Wood, C. & Jakubowicz, D. (1980). The treatment of premenstrual symptoms with mefenamic acid. *British Journal of Obstetrics and Gynaecology* **87**, 627–630.

Wood, C., Larsen, L. & Williams, R. (1979). Menstrual characteristics of 2,343 women attending the Shepherd Foundation. *Australian and New Zealand Journal of Obstetrics and Gynaecology* **19**, 107–110.

Wurtman, J. J., Brzezinski, A., Wurtman, R. J. & Laferrere, B. (1989). Effect of nutrient intake on premenstrual depression. *American Journal of Obstetrics and Gynecology* **161**, 1228–1234.

Young, S. N., Pihl, R. O. & Ervin, F. R. (1988). The effect of altered tryptophan levels on mood and behavior in normal human males. *Clinical Neuropharmacology* **11**, S207–215.

Zimmerman, E. & Parlee, M. B. (1973). Behavioral changes associated with the menstrual cycle: an experimental investigation. *Journal of Applied Social Psychology* **3**, 335–344.